SECONDARY QUALITATIVE DATA ANALYSIS IN THE HEALTH AND SOCIAL SCIENCES

Despite a long history in quantitative research, it is only recently that enthusiasm for secondary analysis of qualitative data has gained momentum across health and social science disciplines. Given that researchers have long known the inordinate amount of time and energy invested in conducting qualitative research, the appeal of secondary analysis of qualitative data is clear. Involving the use of an existing dataset to answer research questions that are different from those asked in the original study, this method allows researchers to once again make use of their hard-earned qualitative dataset and to listen to their participants' voices to the best of their ability in order to improve care and promote understanding.

As secondary qualitative data analysis continues to evolve, more methodological guidance is needed. This book outlines three approaches to secondary data analysis and addresses the key issues that researchers need to wrestle with, such as ethical considerations, voice, and representation. Intellectual and interpretive hazards that can jeopardize the outcome of these analyses are highlighted and discussed, as are the criteria for assessing their quality and trustworthiness.

Written as a thought-provoking guide for qualitative researchers from across the health and social sciences, this text includes a review of the state of the science in nursing and a number of in-depth illustrative case studies.

Cheryl Tatano Beck is a Distinguished Professor at the University of Connecticut, USA, with a joint appointment in the School of Nursing and the School of Medicine.

SECONDARY QUALITATIVE DATA ANALYSIS IN THE HEALTH AND SOCIAL SCIENCES

Cheryl Tatano Beck

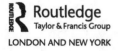

Routledge
Taylor & Francis Group

LONDON AND NEW YORK

First published 2019
by Routledge
2 Park Square, Milton Park, Abingdon, Oxon OX14 4RN

and by Routledge
52 Vanderbilt Avenue, New York, NY 10017

Routledge is an imprint of the Taylor & Francis Group, an informa business

© 2019 Cheryl Tatano Beck

British Library Cataloguing-in-Publication Data
A catalogue record for this book is available from the British Library

Library of Congress Cataloging-in-Publication Data
A catalog record for this book has been requested.

ISBN: 978-1-138-29823-1 (hbk)
ISBN: 978-1-138-29827-9 (pbk)
ISBN: 978-1-315-09875-3 (ebk)

Typeset in Bembo
by codeMantra

This book is dedicated to my husband, Chuck, and my children, Lisa and Curt, for all your love and unwavering support throughout my academic career.

CONTENTS

TABLES AND FIGURES

Tables

Figures

1

INTRODUCTION

In 2004, Heaton published the first book on secondary qualitative analysis. It was groundbreaking. Since then, no other book has been published on the topic. Corti, Van den Eynden, Bishop, and Wollard (2014) have published a related book, *Managing and Sharing Research Data: A Guide to Good Practice*, which addressed effective data management as an essential precondition for high quality reusable data. This current book is the first one published in 15 years since Heaton's book on secondary qualitative data analysis. This book consists of 13 chapters, including this introductory chapter. In this chapter, the outline of the book is presented. A summary of what each chapter addresses is included here, so readers are familiarized with the scope of the book.

Chapter 2 focuses on the history of secondary qualitative data analysis. It began in 1962 when Glaser stressed that secondary analysis should not be limited to quantitative data. He was a proponent of the value that secondary analysis can have for qualitative data. In the early 1990s, U.S. and Canadian researchers and sociologists in the United Kingdom began publishing on the benefits and concerns of secondary qualitative analysis. Different typologies of these analyses were created by Hinds, Vogel, and Clarke-Steffen (1997), Thorne (1994), and Heaton (2004). In 2004, Heaton published the first book on reusing qualitative data. Ten years later, Corti et al. published their book on archiving qualitative data.

In Chapter 3, the advantages and challenges of secondary qualitative analysis are described. Since qualitative research is so time-consuming, what a benefit it is to maximize the use of a dataset to answer new research questions relevant to the phenomenon originally studied. Secondary qualitative analysis can extend the larger context of the primary results. Researchers can reuse primary datasets to reduce participant burden without needing to recruit additional participants. Hazards of secondary qualitative data are also addressed in this chapter. Epistemological and methodological challenges, such as the concern that secondary analysts may not have been present during the original data collection and analysis, are addressed. Secondary analysts are not privy to the insider's experience and may be liable to making incorrect interpretations of the primary dataset. Representational problems of sampling and voice are also described, along with the methodological issues of the fit between the data and the methods in the original study with the new research questions of the secondary analysts.

Chapter 4 concentrates on long-term management of qualitative datasets, namely archiving. Corti et al. (2014) included qualitative archiving as an important part of the research data life cycle. Benefits and challenges of archiving qualitative data are addressed. An example of one benefit is the ability to improve the methodological rigor among qualitative researchers. One of the challenges is anonymizing qualitative datasets. Included in this chapter are the results of studies assessing researchers' attitudes towards qualitative archiving.

Chapter 5 targets ethical concerns of both conducting secondary qualitative analysis and archiving qualitative datasets. Informed consent, confidentiality, and anonymization are key ethical issues. Best practices for anonymizing a qualitative text are identified, along with standard protections of qualitative data in repositories. This chapter includes an example of anonymizing a qualitative dataset for archiving sensitive issues with elusive populations.

Chapter 6 addresses the process involved in actually conducting a secondary qualitative data analysis. Three typologies of secondary qualitative analysis are presented in chronological order. These include Thorne's (1994), Hinds et al.'s (1997), and Heaton's (2004) typologies. Examples of secondary analyses using these typologies from various disciplines are presented to illustrate these typologies. The remainder of the chapter describes steps in conducting this analysis, starting with the research question and ending with archiving the dataset.

International qualitative data archives in the United Kingdom, the United States, Europe, and Australia are highlighted in Chapter 7. The chapter begins with the research data life cycle, which extends the research process beyond just disseminating research findings. Data repository guidelines are covered. Interdisciplinary examples of published secondary qualitative analyses from data obtained from archives are explored in this chapter.

Metaphor analysis is a valuable approach to secondary qualitative data analysis available to secondary analysts. This analysis is the focus of Chapter 8, where two approaches to metaphor analysis are covered: Metaphor Identification Procedure (Pragglejaz Group, 2007) and Steger's (2007) Three-step Metaphor Analysis. The three metaphor analyses I have conducted using my own primary datasets are described to illustrate qualitative secondary analysis using this approach.

In Chapter 9, the use of secondary qualitative data analysis for theory development takes center stage. In 1988, Thorne and Robinson alerted researchers to the use of secondary analysis of multiple qualitative datasets for theory development. Morse (2001) called for secondary analysis of multiple qualitative studies to provide incremental evidence for theory development. In 2017, Morse developed theoretical coalescence as a method of combining qualitative studies to create a higher-level theory. This chapter ends with an example of theoretical coalescence using my own program of research on traumatic childbirth.

Qualitative scholars have a responsibility to prepare the next generation of researchers. Teaching approaches for secondary qualitative data analysis are examined in Chapter 10. Three examples of teaching assignments I have used with my PhD students in my qualitative research methods courses at the University of Connecticut are detailed. The chapter ends by highlighting the U.K. Data Service as an example of a qualitative archive that provides excellent teaching resources for faculty who want to instruct their students in secondary qualitative analysis.

In Chapter 11, general guidelines for writing and publishing secondary qualitative analyses are detailed. An outline for the structure of a secondary qualitative analysis journal article is included. The challenges involved in writing up this type of analysis are identified, and helpful hints to address these challenges are presented. Examples from secondary qualitative analyses I have published are included to illustrate approaches I have used.

Chapter 12 summarizes a literature review that I conducted on secondary qualitative analysis in one discipline, namely nursing. In this review, 274 secondary qualitative analyses were included. Trends and limitations in the reporting of these studies were noted, and recommendations were made.

The final chapter, Chapter 13, looks at the exciting future directions in secondary qualitative data analysis with the hope of further expanding the use of secondary qualitative analysis for theory development and policy development. Recommendations are made for education, publication, ethical issues, and qualitative data archiving.

References

Corti, L., Van den Eynden, V., Bishop, L., & Woollard, M. (2014). *Managing and sharing research data: A guide to good practice*. Los Angeles, CA: Sage Publications.

Heaton, J. (2004). *Reworking qualitative data*. Thousand Oaks, CA: Sage Publications.

Hinds, P. S., Vogel, R. J., & Clarke-Steffen, L. (1997). The possibilities and pitfalls of doing a secondary analysis of a qualitative data set. *Qualitative Health Research, 7*, 408–424.

Morse, J. M. (2001). Qualitative verification: Building evidence by extending basic findings. In J. M. Morse (Ed.), *The nature of qualitative evidence* (pp. 203–220). Thousand Oaks, CA: Sage Publication.

Morse, J. M. (2017). Theoretical coalescence. In J. M. Morse (Ed.), *Analyzing and conceptualizing the theoretical foundations of nursing* (pp. 647–651). New York: Springer Publishing Company.

Pragglejaz Group. (2007). MIP: A method for identifying metaphorically used words in discourse. *Metaphor and Symbol, 22*, 1–39.

Steger, T. (2007). The stories metaphors tell: Metaphors as a tool to describe tacit aspects in narrative. *Field Methods, 19*, 3–23.

Thorne, S. (1994). Secondary analysis in qualitative research: Issues and implications. In J. M. Morse (Ed.), *Critical issues in qualitative research methods* (pp. 263–279). Thousand Oaks, CA: Sage Publications.

2

HISTORY OF SECONDARY QUALITATIVE DATA ANALYSIS

In this chapter, the history of secondary qualitative analysis is described, starting with Glaser in 1962. In the 1990s, sociologists in the United Kingdom and nurse researchers in Canada and the United States contributed early publications on secondary qualitative analysis. From 2000 onward, publications on the reuse of qualitative data have increased substantially. In 2004, Heaton published the first and only book on secondary qualitative data analysis. *The Forum: Qualitative Social Research* is an online journal which has taken the lead on publishing issues devoted to qualitative secondary analysis. Ten years after Heaton's book, Corti, Van den Eymden, Bishop, and Woollard (2014) published their book on archiving data. Bishop (2016) published a chapter on secondary analysis of qualitative data in *Qualitative research: Issues of theory, method and practice.*

Glaser (1962) called man "a data gathering animal" (p. 74). He suggested secondary analysis as a strategy for using the data researchers gather. Secondary analysis is "the study of specific problems through analysis of existing data which were originally collected for other purposes" (Glaser, 1963, p. 11). He stressed that secondary analysis should not be limited to quantitative data.

> The emphasis on survey data neglects other kinds of data, particularly field data, and hence limits the potential use of secondary analysis. This research strategy can be applied to almost any qualitative data however small its amount and whatever the degree of prior analysis.
>
> *(Glaser 1963, p. 11)*

Various types of qualitative data from interviews, field notes, and observation notes can be fruitfully reanalyzed. He went on to state that qualitative researchers may be delighted to have their data, buried in file cabinets for a long time, reanalyzed from a different point of view. Glaser called for tapping past research for its relevance to solving present problems.

Glaser (1962) identified the initial phase in secondary analysis as focusing on the researcher questioning the comparability of the primary data. If the populations included in the primary research and present situation are somewhat the same, the qualitative researcher can determine the characteristics of the original sample and make specific comparisons. If the past sample is not totally a fit, the researcher may have the option of a subgroup. When comparing past problems and results with present problems, secondary researchers are free of the original researcher's purposes. Glaser purported that it doesn't matter if the past problem is similar to the present problem. As long as the data are compatible in regards to population and situation, the secondary analysts can reuse the data according to the specific current problem. He said this is the very essence of secondary analysis. Secondary analysts can take the data to its limits for their own purposes. Back in 1962, Glaser also suggested the option of secondary analysts combining the original dataset with new data to fill in gaps in the past data. Glaser identified other benefits of secondary analysis, such as "economies," which included it being a less expensive process and economy in time since secondary analysis can be accomplished faster than having to collect data.

West and Oldfather (1995) labeled their secondary analysis of qualitative research "pooled case comparison," which begins with raw data. They proposed that their method differed from other comparative methods that start with interpretive findings, such as a meta-ethnography. Their pooled case comparison begins by setting aside the categories and themes from prior analyses. As they stated, the new analysis begins with a "clean slate." West and Oldfather, however, labeled their pooled case comparison as primary data analysis. When reuse of any dataset started with interpreted findings, they called this secondary data analysis, which is the opposite of terms used in the literature. West and Oldfather (1995) stressed that there is an advantage to researchers who were involved in these studies conducting a pooled case comparison rather than using a qualitative data bank. This advantage addressed the deeper knowledge of the context from which the data were obtained. Heshusius (1994) believed that "participatory knowing" cannot be reached through the eyes of even the most interested researchers if they had not been present during the original research.

Social Research Update is published by the Department of Sociology, University of Surrey, and in the 1990s, articles on secondary qualitative data analysis were published there. Corti, Foster, and Thompson (1995) outlined the aims of Qualitative Data Archival Resource Centre (Qualidata). The establishment of Qualidata at the University of Essex was a major breakthrough in archiving qualitative data. At that time, Qualidata was supported by the Economic and Social Resource Council (ESRC) located at the University of Essex in its Sociology Department. The mission of Qualidata was to locate and assess qualitative datasets, and then arrange for their deposit in public archives. Disseminating information about available qualitative datasets and encouraging their reuse were

Qualidata's main aims. At this time, it did not archive qualitative data but arranged for their deposit in appropriate public archive repositories.

Sociologists in the United Kingdom and nurse researchers in Canada and the United States took the lead in the early publications on qualitative secondary analysis. After Glaser's (1962, 1963) call for the use of secondary analysis not only with quantitative data but also with qualitative data, Thorne (1994) published the first article on qualitative secondary analysis. She argued for the potential contribution of secondary analysis of time-intensive qualitative datasets. She acknowledged some of its hazards and then went on to discuss issues in secondary analysis, such as the fit between the datasets and the research questions. In this groundbreaking publication, Thorne identified five discrete types of research involved in secondary qualitative analysis: analytic expansion, retrospective interpretation, armchair induction, amplified sampling, and cross-validation.

In 1997, three articles were published by nurse researchers. Sandelowski (1997) spoke to secondary analysis as a way to enhance the utility of qualitative research. She wrote that researchers "have become inveterate data collectors, have been imbued with the idea that research means collecting new data" (p. 129). She called for supporting innovative treatments of qualitative data to yield new, useful knowledge.

Hinds, Vogel, and Clarke-Steffen (1997) addressed the possibilities and pitfalls of doing secondary analysis of a qualitative dataset. They developed a set of four different types of secondary analysis depending on whether a different unit of analysis was used, whether only a subset of cases or the entire dataset was reanalyzed, or whether new data were also collected. Hinds et al. (1997) provided an example of an assessment tool that focused on criteria for use in secondary analysis of qualitative datasets. Criteria for determining the general quality of the original study dataset and the fit of the secondary research question were included in the tool. Hinds and colleagues also provided an example of an amended consent form for permission to use data for secondary analysis.

Other early proponents of secondary qualitative data analysis included Szabo and Strang (1997). They described the use of secondary analysis with their study on family caregivers of relatives with dementia. Their new research question fit well with the primary dataset. The purpose of the primary study was to explore the meaning and achievements of respite for caregivers of relatives with dementia. Their secondary study focused on how caregivers' perceived control helped them to manage their caregiving for family members with dementia.

Another publication in the 1990s was again by Thorne (1998); in it, she addressed two specific concerns in qualitative secondary analysis: ethical and representational issues. Hammersley (1997) added to this initial discussion of qualitative secondary analysis the need to create qualitative data archives. Hammersley identified two main purposes in archiving qualitative data. First, it would facilitate assessment of the validity of the primary studies, and second, it would increase the scope of secondary analysis. Corti and Thompson (1998) published a paper alerting researchers to the mission of Qualidata.

Mauthner, Parry, and Backett-Milburn (1998) discussed their own experiences revisiting their data and the implications of researchers' reflexivity in archiving and reusing qualitative data. They warned that "if researchers generate new substantive findings and theories from old qualitative data, without attending to the epidemiological issues, they are being 'naively realist'" (p. 743).

Heaton (1998) published an article on secondary analysis of qualitative data in *Social Research Update*. She outlined the forms of this type of analysis and key ethical and methodological issues involved with it. Heaton (2000) conducted a literature review on qualitative secondary analysis studies in health and social care research. Sixty-five studies were located, 51 of which were conducted by authors in North America. Twelve of the remaining studies were conducted by researchers in the United Kingdom, one from Sweden, and one was a Canadian-Swedish study. Thirty-six of the 65 studies were carried out by researchers who reused their own original datasets. Twenty secondary analyses were conducted by a mix of one or more researchers from the original study in collaboration with researchers who were not involved with the primary study. Fourteen percent ($n = 9$) of the secondary analyses were carried out by researchers who had no direct knowledge or experience with the primary study. Heaton (2000) also reported that in 48 studies, single datasets were reused. Two datasets were used in 14 studies, and three studies combined three or more databases. The databases ranged from less than 10 to more than 200 interviews. In approximately half of the secondary studies, the original datasets were reused in total; in the other half, a subset of the database was used. In nine of the studies, additional new data were collected and added to the preexisting dataset. Heaton (2000) identified five types of secondary analysis used in the studies included in her literature review: supra analysis, supplementary analysis, reanalysis, amplified analysis, and assorted analysis.

In Germany, Mruck (2000) initiated the *Forum: Qualitative Social Research* to promote online resources for qualitative researchers. Since then, this online journal has devoted three complete issues to qualitative secondary analysis and archiving. The first issue was published in 2000 and was dedicated to "Text. Archive. Re-Analysis." Forty-six authors in various disciplines from 13 different countries discussed in 27 articles their experiences with documenting, archiving, accessing, and reanalyzing qualitative data.

Heaton (2004) identified three main modes of qualitative secondary analysis: formal data sharing, informal data sharing, and self-collected data. In formal data sharing, researchers access datasets housed in public or institutional archives and reuse them. For informal data sharing, there are a number of possibilities. The original researchers may choose to share their data with other researchers who may have had some involvement in the primary study, while others may have had no prior involvement. The original researchers may or may not be involved with the secondary analysis. With self-collected data, the original researchers reuse their own datasets. Another option here is for multiple original researchers to combine their datasets and reanalyze these data together.

One of the *Forum: Qualitative Social Research* special issues in 2005 (Vol. 6, No. 1) focused on the potential and the problems of secondary qualitative analysis. The three sections in this issue included (1) issues of context, (2) approaches to reuse: asking new questions of old data, and (3) procedures for archiving qualitative data: confidentiality and technical issues. The second issue of this online journal (Vol. 6, No. 2) in 2005, devoted to secondary qualitative analysis, focused on the why and the how of archiving qualitative data. The situations in different European countries were described (France, Great Britain, and Germany).

Corti (2012) reviewed some of the major issues she had encountered working with a national data archiving organization since 1995. She discussed four developments in data archiving in social research from 2006 to 2011: new approaches to archiving qualitative data, providing safe access to disclosed datasets, institutional data archiving initiatives, and new data types. Under new approaches, Corti identified metadata standards for qualitative research for formally describing the data. She also discussed the ongoing debate of capturing context related to the loss of the primary researchers' "being there" as secondary analysts try to reuse the data. Last, Corti (2012) described new data types, such as Internet surveys, blogs, and chat rooms, that provide a challenge for archiving as the data landscape rapidly changes. Another new type of data for archives is "enhanced publication," which provides an interactive publication where readers can view the actual data excerpts.

In reviewing a decade of secondary qualitative data reuse primarily in the United Kingdom, Bishop and Kuula-Luumi (2017) provided evidence of the growth of data reuse. They used downloads of archived data collections held at data repositories and publication citations as sources for their review. Some factors enabling this upswing in the number of secondary qualitative analyses included an increase in data repositories being established within universities, improved infrastructure, and services that facilitate access to data archives.

New creative ways to share qualitative data are being published in the literature. Stamm (2018), for example, described how organized research communities, which consist of small groups of researchers, can share primary data with each other. She calls this a hybrid form of data sharing which is placed between informal sharing through individual researchers collaborating with each other and institutional qualitative archives.

Summary

As we can see, publications on secondary qualitative data analysis began in the 1990s. From 2000 onward, interest in reuse of qualitative data has grown substantially. Issues in one journal, *Forum: Qualitative Social Research* (2000, 2005), were devoted to qualitative secondary data analysis. In 2004, Heaton published the first book on *Reworking Qualitative Data*. Ten years later, Corti et al. (2014) published a book focusing on managing, sharing, and archiving data.

In the literature published during this time period, researchers debated concerns over reanalyzing qualitative data. The main controversial issues being debated were ethical, philosophical, and legal issues; the fit of the datasets to new research questions; and the problem of secondary researchers not having collected the data and therefore "not being there." While acknowledging that there are some dangers with this type of analysis, there is growing evidence of the awareness among qualitative researchers of the value of secondary qualitative data analysis. There is an accelerated emergence of secondary qualitative data analysis as a viable research method. In the next chapter, the benefits of, as well as the challenges in, conducting secondary qualitative data analyses are explored.

References

Bishop, L. (2016). Secondary analysis of qualitative data. In D. Silverman (Ed.), *Qualitative research: Issues of theory, method and practice* (4th ed., pp. 395–411). London: Sage.

Bishop, L., & Kuula-Luumi, A. (2017). Revisiting qualitative data reuse: A decade on. *Sage Open.* doi:10.1177/2158244016685136

Corti, L. (2012). Recent development in archiving social research. *International Journal of Social Research Methodology, 15,* 281–290.

Corti, L., Foster, J., & Thompson, P. (1995). Archiving qualitative research data. *Social Research Update.* Issue 10, University of Surrey.

Corti, L., & Thompson, P. (1998). Are you sitting on your qualitative data? Qualidata's mission. *International Journal of Social Research Methodology, 1,* 85–89.

Corti, L., Van den Eynden, V., Bishop, L., & Woollard, M. (2014). *Managing and sharing research data: A guide to good practice.* Los Angeles, CA: Sage Publications.

Glaser, B. G. (1962). Secondary analysis: A strategy for the use of knowledge from research elsewhere. *Social Problems, 10,* 70–74.

Glaser, B. G. (1963). Retreading research materials: The use of secondary analysis by the independent researcher. *The American Behavioral Scientist, 6,* 11–14.

Hammersley, M. (1997). Qualitative data archiving: Some reflections in its prospects and problems. *Sociology, 31,* 131–142.

Heaton, J. (1998, October). Secondary analysis of qualitative data. *Social Research Update.* Issue 22, University of Surrey.

Heaton, J. (2000). *Secondary analysis of qualitative data: A review of the literature.* York, England: Social Policy Research Unit (SPRU), University of York.

Heaton, J. (2004). *Reworking qualitative data.* Thousand Oaks, CA: Sage.

Heshusius, L. (1994). Freeing ourselves from objectivity: Managing subjectivity or turning toward a participatory mode of consciousness? *Educational Researcher, 23,* 15–23.

Hinds, P. S., Vogel, R. J., & Clarke-Steffen, L. (1997). The possibilities and pitfalls of doing a secondary analysis of a qualitative data set. *Qualitative Health Research, 7,* 408–424.

Mauthner, N. S., Parry, O., & Backett-Milburn, K. (1998). The data are out there, or are they? Implications for archiving and revisiting qualitative data. *Sociology, 32,* 733–745.

Mruck, K. (2000). Qualitative research networking: FQS as an Example. *Forum: Qualitative Social Research, 1*(3), Art. 34. Retrieved from http://nbn-resolving.de/urn:nbn:de:0114-fqs0003346

Sandelowski, M. (1997). "To be of use": Enhancing the utility of qualitative research. *Nursing Outlook, 45,* 125–132.

Stamm, I. (2018). Organized communities as a hybrid from of data sharing: Experiences from the Global STEP Project. *Forum Qualitative Social Research,* *19*(1), Art. 16, doi:10.17169/fqs-19.1.2885

Szabo, V., & Strang, V. (1997). Secondary analysis of qualitative data. *Advances in Nursing Science, 20,* 66–74.

Thorne, S. (1994). Secondary analysis in qualitative research: Issues and implications. In J. M. Morse (Ed.), *Critical issues in qualitative research methods* (pp. 263–279). Thousand Oaks, CA: Sage Publications.

Thorne, S. (1998). Ethical and representational issues in qualitative secondary analysis. *Qualitative Health Research, 8,* 574–555.

West, J., & Oldfather, P. (1995). Pooled case comparison: An innovation for cross-case study. *Qualitative Inquiry, 1,* 452–464.

3
BENEFITS AND CONCERNS OF SECONDARY QUALITATIVE DATA ANALYSIS

In this chapter, both the advantages and disadvantages of secondary qualitative analysis are presented. First the benefits of secondary qualitative analysis are discussed followed by the concerns regarding this analytic method. Research transparency is discussed as a means to increasing the benefits of secondary qualitative data analysis.

Potential contributions of secondary qualitative analysis

Qualitative research is quite time-consuming, which requires serious commitment to data collecting, such as in face-to-face interviews, participant observation, and transcribing interview data, and then analysis of the volume of data. An advantage to maximizing the use of a qualitative dataset is to answer new, important questions relevant to the phenomenon that was originally studied. The potential exists for secondary qualitative analysis to extend the larger context of research results. It can promote generalizability of qualitative research findings and also salvage data from the original study which had not been completely analyzed (Heaton, 2004). Secondary analysis can provide a means for continuance of older qualitative findings. Researchers can track the progression of the new trends and knowledge by reusing the older datasets for comparison. Data from original research can be reexamined in the light of different insights from others' research. Gadamer (1988) pointed out that historical consciousness toward data may help to clarify prejudices and increase the potential for understanding phenomena.

At a time when research funding is exceedingly difficult to secure, secondary analysis is cost effective. It provides maximum use of the original dataset. As funders are beginning to require archiving of data, reuse of data maximizes the benefit of publicly funded research for the good of the public. Additional benefits of secondary qualitative analysis target the development of qualitative theory. Using raw data in secondary analysis, instead of relying on themes or coding from published qualitative studies, increases the scope, abstraction, and generalizability of theory development (Morse, 2018). Secondary analysis of qualitative datasets also has the potential to contribute to health policy formulation (Ziebland & Hunt, 2014). Policy makers often have time constraints and do not have the luxury of conducting research to help guide their policymaking. This can result in the valuable voices of patients from being excluded from the development of the health policy. Secondary qualitative data analysis can remedy this and allow patient experiences to inform policy decision making.

Secondary analysis of qualitative data allows continued research on topics related to a specific population without needing recruitment of any additional participants. Both quantitative and qualitative researchers need to be cognizant of reducing participant burden. Secondary analysis can also facilitate more research with marginalized, vulnerable populations who may be difficult to recruit in research studies. An example of this benefit in a hard-to-reach population is provided by Owens, Hansford, Sharkey, and Ford (2016), who conducted a secondary qualitative data analysis of the needs and fears of young people presenting at emergency departments following an act of self-harm. The original study was an online discussion forum during the summer of 2009 (Owens et al., 2015). The full cohort in the primary study included 77 young people. In this secondary analysis 31 of these participants were included. Four themes emerged which corresponded to phases of the young person's journey to and through the emergency department: influences on the decision to attend or avoid, feelings on arrival, perceptions of treatment and care, and consequences of perceived negative treatment.

In order to fully reap the benefits of secondary qualitative analysis Moravcsik (2014) called for research transparency. He termed this the methodological revolution in qualitative research. In research transparency researchers make the essential components of their studies visible for other researchers. He identified three dimensions of research transparency:

1. Data transparency allows readers access to the data and the evidence that researchers used to support researchers' empirical results. It helps readers evaluate if the data were analyzed correctly.
2. Analytic transparency provides the ability to review information regarding data analysis. The interpretive process the researcher used to support claims is accessible to readers.
3. Production transparency gives readers access to the methods by which the researcher chose pieces of data from the entire body of the interview. Since the findings only represent a subset of the data relevant to the research question, there can be danger of selection bias. Data transparency can help prevent this.

Moravcsik (2014) advocates for active citation which is an applicable tool for facilitating qualitative research transparency. Active citation includes any citation in a scholarly paper, article, or book chapter that supports a contestable empirical claim is hyperlinked to an excerpt from the original source and an annotation explaining how that excerpt supports the empirical claim, located in a 'transparency appendix' attached to the document.

(Moravcsik, 2014, p. 48)

He described the entries for each citation (p. 50):

1. A copy of the full citation
2. An excerpt from the source, presumptively at least 50–100 words
3. An annotation explaining how the source supports the claim being made
4. Optionally, an outside link to and/or a scan of the full source.

Hazards within secondary qualitative analysis

There are a number of hazards that may jeopardize the quality of secondary qualitative analysis (Thorne, 1994). Qualitative findings are never free from the perspective of the researcher. Since bias will exist in datasets along with interpretive methods used to analyze these data, the potential exists in secondary analysis to exaggerate the impact of those biases. Specific features of the primary dataset may not be obvious to the secondary researcher. The original researcher may be privy to a multitude of contexts that influenced the direction of data collection and analysis. The primary researcher's role in constructing the findings may be challenging to reconstruct the tacit understandings at a later date. Bishop (2016) noted, however, that insights from data rely not only on the primary researcher "being there" but also on the analytical abilities of the secondary analyst.

A fundamental premise of qualitative research is the critical relationship between the researcher and the participants. Secondary analysts lack this crucial relationship and can be liable of making an incorrect interpretation of the primary dataset (Cliggett, 2013). Thorne (1998) highlighted the issue of fidelity: "Distance between the original data source and the analyst poses threats to fidelity in the interpretation of findings beyond those presumed in the primary research" (p. 551). Simmons, Nelson, and Simonsohn (2011) term the culprit "researcher degrees of freedom. In the course of collecting and analyzing data, researchers have many decisions to make: Should more data be collected? Should some observations be excluded?" (p. 1359). Thorne (2013) described this problem as the original research "reveals the handprint of the researcher who has played a role in co-creating it" (p. 395). The results of the original study were shaped both overtly and covertly by the researcher. Secondary analysts who were not involved in the primary researcher are not privy to the insider's experience. A concern for secondary analysts can occur when the original research was on sensitive topics. Secondary analysts did not collect the data and they might have strong emotional responses to reading the interview transcripts or listening to the tape recordings which they had not expected (Hinds, Vogel, & Clarke-Steffen, 1997).

Other concerns with secondary qualitative analysis include representational problems having to do with sampling and voice (Thorne, 1998). Due to the typical but appropriate small sample size in qualitative research, one issue is related to the degree that any qualitative study can represent more than the participants who comprised the sample. Secondary qualitative analysis could lead to conditions which exaggerate any representational problems of the primary research. Another hazard is what Thorne (1994) called "lazy" research where primary datasets are reanalyzed multiple times.

Voice is another issue that secondary analysts need to contend with. Thorne (1998) warned that

> because the sociopolitical consciousness of a group may undergo collective change, interpretations that would have been acceptable to members at one time may not be understood the same way at a later point .... Thus the obligation of the secondary analyst in the context of politically sensitive health knowledge may extend as far as negotiation with those who hold social credibility as advocates for particular voices within society at the time of the secondary research.
>
> *(p. 553)*

The fit between the data and the methods by which the primary dataset was constructed is another major challenge for secondary qualitative analysis. Secondary analysts need to understand the impact of the methodology used in the original study and determine if it is amenable to secondary analysis. Thorne (2013) warns that since aspects of a qualitative study may be idiosyncratic to the primary researchers, "assumptions based on general methodological claims by the original researcher may be somewhat misleading" (p. 395). Depending on the interview technique used, certain themes may or may not have been investigated. Thorne went on to caution that "interpretation dependent on the qualitative equivalent of intensity or frequency of thematic material can be seriously confounded by misinterpretations of the design and implementation of the data collection process" (p. 395).

Hinds et al. (1997) addressed the issue of missing data when determining the fit of the original dataset to the secondary research question. These authors described the problem of missing data in qualitative studies when the primary researchers explored an issue in one interview but not all of the interviews. Perhaps this occurred in the original study as the researchers narrowed the study's scope and refined the interview question. When a phenomenon was not uniformly investigated in the original study, the fit between that dataset and the secondary analysts' research questions may not match.

The currency of the data can be another problem with the fit of the primary dataset to a new research question. It may no longer be appropriate for the secondary study's research question. Greater distance between the primary study and the secondary analysis can make the secondary analysis more problematic. Last, Bishop

(2016) cautions that reusing qualitative archives may not always be faster than collecting original data. The time required to search, find, and access the appropriate archived data that fit your research question can also be time intensive.

In summary both the advantages and disadvantages of secondary qualitative analysis were discussed in this chapter. "Secondary qualitative analysis holds tremendous promise to the scholar seeking to do justice to the investments of the original inquiries and to follow the logical threads of an investigative promise" (Thorne, 2013, p. 397). In the next chapter, the debate over archiving qualitative data will be the focus.

References

Bishop, L. (2016). Secondary analysis of qualitative data. In D. Silverman (Ed.), *Qualitative research: Issues of theory, method, and practice* (pp. 395–411). London: Sage.

Cliggett, L. (2013). Qualitative data archiving in the digital age: Strategies for data preservation and sharing. *The Qualitative Report, 18*, 1–11.

Gadamer, H. G. (1988). On the circle of understanding. In J. M. Connally & T. Kentner (Trans. & Eds.), *Hermeneutics versus science? Three German Essays.* Notre Dame, IN: University of Notre Dame Press.

Heaton, J. (2004). *Reworking qualitative data.* Thousand Oaks, CA: Sage Publications.

Hinds, P. S., Vogel, R. J., & Clarke-Steffen, L. (1997). The possibilities and pitfalls of doing a secondary analysis of a qualitative data set. *Qualitative Health Research, 7*, 408–424.

Moravcsik, A. (2014). Transparency: The revolution in qualitative research. *Political Science & Politics, 47*, 48–53.

Morse, J. M. (2018). Theoretical coalescence: A method to develop qualitative theory. *Nursing Research, 67*, 177–187.

Owens, C., Hansford, L., Sharkey, S., & Ford, T. (2016). Needs and fears of young people presenting at accident and emergency departments following an act of self-harm: Secondary analysis of qualitative data. *The British Journal of Psychiatry, 208*, 286–291.

Owens, C., Sharkey, S., Smithson, J., Hewis, E., Emmens, T., Ford, T., et al. (2015). Building an online community to promote communication and collaborative learning between health professional and young people who self-harm: An exploratory study. *Health Expectations, 18*, 81–94.

Simmons, J. P., Nelson, L. D., & Simonsohn, U. (2011). False-positive psychology: Undisclosed flexibility in data collection and analysis allows presenting anything as significant. *Psychological Science, 22*, 1359–1366.

Thorne, S. (1994). Secondary analysis in qualitative research: Issues and implications. In J. M. Morse (Ed.), *Critical issues in qualitative research methods* (pp. 263–279). London: Sage.

Thorne, S. (1998). Ethical and representational issues in qualitative secondary analysis. *Qualitative Health Research, 8*, 547–555.

Thorne, S. (2013). Secondary qualitative data analysis. In C. T. Beck (Ed.), *Routledge international handbook of qualitative nursing research* (pp. 393–404). New York: Routledge.

Ziebland, S., & Hunt, K. (2014). Using secondary analysis of qualitative data of patient experiences of health care to inform health services research and policy. *Journal of Health Services Research & Policy, 19*, 177–182.

4

DEBATE OVER ARCHIVING QUALITATIVE DATA

Just as with conducting a secondary qualitative analysis, archiving qualitative data also has benefits along with concerns. Chapter 4 addresses both of these issues. Researchers' attitudes toward sharing and archiving qualitative data have been studied and these findings are described. An example of one benefit discussed here is the ability to improve methodological rigor among qualitative researchers. Roller and Lavrakas's (2017) Total Quality Framework and its four major components are identified in this chapter. One of the challenges in archiving that is discussed in this chapter is anonymizing qualitative datasets. An example of qualitative archiving in Poland is presented to close the chapter.

Benefits of qualitative data sharing and archiving

Data sharing can bring visibility and evidence to support the findings in a primary dataset. Due to the page constraints in journals, when the primary researcher is publishing the results, only a limited number of quotes and actual data are permitted. The complete dataset can be made available in an archive. This helps the trustworthiness of the analysis in the primary research (Antes, Walsh, Strait, Hudson-Vitale, & Dubois, 2018). Education of our future generation of researchers will also be enhanced by having archived datasets to practice analyzing qualitative data under the mentorship of faculty. Professors teaching qualitative research methods courses to PhD students can use archived datasets in their classes for assignments.

More and more funding agencies are beginning to require plans for archiving of data when submitting grants. This would support compliance with funders' requirements. In the previous chapter the benefits of secondary qualitative analysis were discussed. If qualitative datasets are archived, this will facilitate secondary qualitative analysis. Secondary analysts will have other options besides informal, non-archived datasets to use. Primary researchers who archive their qualitative dataset can reap the benefits of an increased citation rate. Archiving qualitative data will also support meta-syntheses. Meta-synthesizers will have the complete dataset and will not have to settle for using just the published findings in articles.

Currently, if qualitative researchers want to check the results of their study with that of another study, they often have to conduct research themselves on the phenomenon. By archiving, data will be available and can decrease the costs of replication studies. This is especially important for mixed methods studies where the qualitative strand, which is often the lower priority strand, results in the unavailability of the data as a smaller portion of the article is devoted to the qualitative data (Elman, Kapiszewski, & Vinuela, 2010).

Roller and Lavrakas (2017) believe the greatest benefit of sharing qualitative data is the opportunity to raise the bar on methodological rigor among the qualitative research community. Transparency via thick description assists collaborations among researchers to continually improve upon each other's method and in turn yield more insights into human experiences. What should be shared by qualitative researchers when sharing their data? Roller and Lavrakas (2017) developed the Total Quality Framework (TQF), which consisted of four major components: credibility, analyzability, transparency, and usefulness. Credibility addresses two issues: (1) how representative the sample is of the target population (scope) and (2) how well the data were gathered. Analyzability focuses on (1) data processing—what was done with the data and how they were transcribed—and (2) verification—how results and conclusions were verified.

Credibility: scope

- Clear definition of the target population.
- Description of the list chosen to represent the target population and how participants were chosen from the list.
- Strategies used to gain access to study participants including why some participants decided not to be in the study.
- Describe sample size and rationale for that number.

Credibility: data gathering

- Description of phenomenon being studied.
- Provision of data collection instruments. If newly developed, provide pilot testing data.
- Description of modes of data collection.
- Information on who was in the research team and their qualifications and training.
- Identification of any bias or inconsistency during data collection.
- Description of any possible participant effects that may have biased the data.

- De-identified data.
- Reflexive journal written during the study after de-identification.

Analyzability: data processing

- Description of persons who transcribed the data, their qualifications and training, and the monitoring procedures put in place to oversee the quality of their work.
- Description of how transcriptions were done, including directions to transcriptionists.
- Description of other forms of data, such as videos, that were included.
- Description of how and why the unit of analysis was chosen.
- Description of how codes were devised and the coding process.
- Description of who the coders were, their qualifications and the monitoring of their work.
- Explanation of how meaningful categories were identified.
- Explanation of the rationale and method for determining themes.
- Explanation of how the interpretations and implications were created.

Analyzability: verification

- Description of how verification was done (peer debriefings) triangulation, negative cases.
- Description of how the findings from the verification were used.

Roller and Lavrakas asked researchers to consider if there are unique data-sharing issues associated with different qualitative research designs such as grounded theory and phenomenology.

Concerns associated with qualitative data sharing and archiving

Preparing a qualitative dataset for archiving is time-consuming. So much is involved in this preparation: anonymizing, transferring dataset in file formats accepted by the repository, producing metadata, and making sure of adequate data documentation (Cliggett, 2013). Removal of both direct and indirect identifiers may be required to ensure participants' anonymity. If important contextual information is deleted, the primary researcher should create a log of these changes to the dataset (Antes et al., 2018). Researchers may not have the skills nor institutional resources to help with data curation.

Concerns over researchers conducting secondary analysis when they did not actually collect the primary data are apparent. Secondary researchers are not privy to context-specific and relationship-dependent information the primary researcher had. Secondary analysts do not have depth of contextual knowledge to make sense of the dataset as the primary data collector had. Dubois, Strait, and Walsh (2017) shared concerns about archiving qualitative data. Reflexivity is definitely limited when a researcher has no role in gathering the data that were analyzed. It is naive to think that secondary analysts will have access to the same level of information as the primary researcher. Dubois and colleagues listed some of their other concerns, such as some forms of anonymization that can be misleading, permission and ownership, confidentiality and harms, and protecting data ownership.

Protecting participants' privacy, confidentiality, and consent are concerns. Worries over the misuse of data in secondary research, especially with vulnerable populations, are also concerns of primary researchers. Alderson (1998) warned that primary researchers and archivists can control who accesses the dataset, however, they cannot guarantee the data will be reused appropriately or sensitively. Richardson and Godfrey (2003) warned that the ethical responsibility and bond between the original researcher and participants are more distant and tenuous for the reader of transcribed interviews.

Regarding sharing and archiving data qualitative researchers are uneasy about the epistemological challenges of using data removed from their contexts of production. Context provides the foundation from which meaning thrives in qualitative research. How context shapes the data themselves raises concerns about archiving and sharing qualitative data. Contextual data can mold the data in one direction or another. Secondary analysis is only as valuable as the information the primary researcher archives on the dataset such as, field notes, codebooks, interview guides, references, etc. (Roller & Lavrakas, 2017).

Earlier in this chapter transparency of qualitative datasets was listed as a benefit of data archiving. It can, however, have a downside. An unintended result of transparency can be to encourage qualitative researchers to engage in self-censorship where they may omit archiving data collected by a method they fear would not be viewed as rigorous or observations that could reflect in an unfavorable light on either themselves or a participant (Elman et al., 2010). Elman and colleagues also described another problem if "share-ability" becomes an overriding criterion by which datasets are judged: qualitative researchers may tend to focus only on contexts in which data can be collected that are easily archived. This could result in researchers' not collecting relevant information.

Another concern focuses on limits to sharing qualitative data. Sometimes interviews are conducted off the record and participants are promised that their data will not be used. Some participants may be unwilling to have their data archived for other researchers to use. Kuula (2011), however, investigated the attitudes of 169 participants from four qualitative studies regarding data archiving and sharing and 98% of the participants allowed their data to be archived.

Cliggett (2013) addressed one barrier to consider regarding archiving and data sharing. This involves the primary researchers' threat of being scooped when not receiving recognition as the author of the primary dataset. Protecting data ownership is an important issue. Travers (2009) warned that secondary analysts can use some data for different purposes than the primary researcher and may even present that researcher in a negative light. Travers also raised concerns about how the diversity of research methods employed by qualitative researchers and how different traditions yield findings within specific theoretical assumptions are not highlighted in teaching guidelines in qualitative data repositories.

Challenges in anonymizing qualitative datasets

For data sharing and archiving there are multiple stages to the process of anonymizing. First is what Saunders, Kitzinger, and Kitzinger (2015) call crude anonymization of the entire transcripts so that they could be entered into the data management system and be shared with the research team. Next comes anonymizing individual data quotes when submitting a manuscript for publication; in essence, creating a smoke screen when necessary. Another round of anonymizing is necessary if archiving of data will occur. Saunders et al. warn that even the first phase of anonymizing is extremely time-consuming and has implications for funding of data sharing. Future funding proposals need to include costs for the time commitment to anonymize the qualitative dataset.

An example of the challenges that face qualitative researchers in anonymizing interview data, especially in highly sensitive contexts, is provided by Saunders et al. (2015). These researchers described the issues they faced in maximizing anonymity in their sample of family members of persons in vegetative and minimally conscious states. They went on to share the elaborate, context-sensitive strategies they used to protect the participants but at the same time preserve the richness of the interview data. Key areas were addressed in anonymizing: people's name, places, religious or cultural background, occupation, family relationships, and other potentially identifying information. Regarding people's names, on occasion, the researchers avoided using the same pseudonym for both of the quotes in order to prevent readers from identifying two data extracts spoken by the same person. In considering religious and cultural backgrounds Saunders et al. (2015) often replaced religion/culture with similar but unrelated terms, such as changing "Hinduism" to "religious faith." At times though it was especially problematic when religion or culture was crucial for a deeper understanding of the data. Sometimes by removing reference to any specific religion, Saunders and colleagues (2015, p. 624) asked themselves "whether we have veered too far, and 'white-washed' the data, 'forfeiting much of the richness yielded' by the study and draining it of its meaning?" Occupation for some interviews was also salient and proved challenging to remove or alter. Whenever the researchers could keep the family relationships, they did, but there were times when they felt it necessary to disguise them. For example, Saunders et al. avoided identifying gay relationships. They struggled, though, because in their attempt to preserve anonymity, they erased some of the experiences of minorities. The minority status of participants predisposed them to being easily identified. When using quotes that could reveal possible identification of minority or atypical relationships, the researchers took extra steps to make sure quotes were presented in isolation from other ones from the same participant. Saunders et al. stressed that anonymizing was a continual working compromise. At times they had to sacrifice the integrity of the data in order to protect anonymity but at other times they may have risked compromising anonymity to maintain data integrity. The researchers shared that they became more skilled at identifying, during an interview, times when potential problems of anonymizing what participants were saying could occur. The researchers were then able to raise these concerns of anonymizing with the interviewee while the interview was still going on.

Researchers' attitudes on archiving qualitative data

Scientists' attitudes and practices of qualitative data sharing have been assessed through surveys, focus groups, and interviews. The first study focused on Australian researchers' views on qualitative archiving where six focus groups with a total of 37 qualitative researchers were held (Broom, Cheshire, & Emmison, 2009). Few of the researchers had any prior experience in qualitative data archiving, but some researchers had archived quantitative data. One common theme that surfaced in all the focus groups was that qualitative research is an art and a relationship. Qualitative research is about special relationships between researchers and their participants where situated narratives are coproduced. Questions were raised concerning how these relationships could be transferred into an archive for different researchers to be able to conduct a meaningful secondary analysis. Archived data were viewed as excluding the all-important unique context of these interactional elements of trust and reciprocity that coproduced the qualitative findings. Focus group members shared their belief that "data become disembodied and disembedded when archived, thereby increasing the likelihood that subsequent researchers would 'misinterpret' those data as a result" (Broom et al., 2009, p. 1170).

Another theme that emerged in the focus group centered on qualitative researchers' belief that no one else could understand their data; the idea of the solitary researcher going it alone. Some focus group members did suggest that there may be a need for a change toward team work. Some felt the solitary researcher could undermine the view of qualitative research as a rigorous method. Tensions were apparent between the "solitary ideal" versus group analysis of data.

"'What's mine is …mine': The protection of rights and intellectual property" (Broom et al., 2009, p. 1173) was the third issue addressed in the focus groups. Concerns over research ethics and data ownership were shared. Qualitative researchers spoke of needing to ensure that the participants' rights and confidentiality were protected. Researchers were also concerned about allowing their own private and personal recollections, such as ethnographic field notes, to become public. The fourth theme involved sharing qualitative data as an ethical imperative. There was debate in the focus group about data ownership. Two of the focus groups viewed data sharing as the responsibility of qualitative researchers to "get participants stories out there." Data are a community resource and should not be just for the individual researchers' own professional interests.

In a national survey conducted in 2008 of Swedish qualitative social scientists' attitudes toward data sharing, 65% of the researchers stated that what prevented them from archiving their data were threats to confidentiality (Carlhed & Alfredsson, 2009). Approximately 50% of the researchers stated that archiving was either never done or very unusual. In Finland in a similar survey 66% of qualitative researchers stated that the lack of informed consent was a major obstacle to archiving their data and 48% reported confidentiality and research ethics were the reasons for not sharing data (Kuula & Borg, 2008).

A nationwide feasibility study on archiving and using secondary qualitative data was conducted in Germany (Medjedović, 2011). It was a joint effort between the "Archive for Life Course Research" and the GESIS Leibniz Institute for the social sciences. A survey was sent to 1,104 qualitative project managers from 1993 or later; the return rate was 39% ($N = 430$). From the 430 respondents, 36 qualitative researchers were invited to be interviewed to explore the issue in more depth. Eighty percent of the researchers were in favor of building an infrastructure for archiving qualitative research in Germany. Approximately 60% of the qualitative project managers in principle were willing to archive their data for secondary analysis by other researchers. When asked if they could imagine conducting secondary analysis in the future themselves, 65% said "yes." Around 60% ($n = 270$) of the researchers stated they had never done secondary analysis of qualitative data. When asked why not, 40% gave no special reason or said that they had no time or resources. Eighty respondents (~20%) said they would not provide their data in principle for other researchers to use. Their major objection (40.8%) dealt with data protection and confidentiality. Career-related self-interest and concerns regarding misuse of data by others also influenced the qualitative project managers to object to sharing their data. Another major argument against archiving was the effort required for preparing the dataset for secondary use.

Example of qualitative archiving in Poland

In Poland the practice of archiving qualitative data has been relatively recent (Niedbalski & S'lezak, 2018). In 2012 the Polish Code of Sociologist Ethics adopted by the Polish Sociological Association included a provision related to data archiving. Point 38 of the code states "Sociologists should popularize the results of their research as much as possible, and if there is such a need, immediately upon completion of their analysis, to provide other researchers with their data through the applied archives and databases" (as cited in Niedbalski & S'lezak, 2018, p. 251). Currently in Poland it is not obligatory nor legally required for researchers to archive their data. Polish researchers raised the issue of a conflict of values: the need to protect the anonymity of their participants versus the need to protect the richness of personal biographical stories as a valuable historical source from being destroyed or lost.

Niedbalski and S'lezak (2018) provided a specific example to illustrate Polish qualitative researchers' concerns about negotiating consent for data archiving with their participants. This example comes from their research with women who provide sex services in escort agencies. When conducting qualitative research with sensitive phenomena like prostitution, consent for archiving can be troublesome or even impossible to obtain. The leaking of information from either audiotapes or transcriptions of the interview data may make their way to unauthorized persons and could be used against these participants, which may be of special concern for these women. Even just requesting permission to archive these data with the women may influence the direction the interview takes or even the possibility the participants will refuse to be interviewed at all.

Another issue regarding obtaining permission for qualitative data archiving concerns when the researcher should make this request (Niedbalski and S'lezak, 2018). If consent is obtained prior to the interview it could result (1) in self-censorship where the participant may avoid talking about certain experiences and/or (2) it could lead to self-presentation where the participants stress experiences that would present them in the best place to be entered into the archive. If the researcher, however, chooses to consent to archiving after the interview is completed, participants may refuse for any part of their interview to be used in the research study.

In summary, this chapter addressed both the benefits as well as researchers' concerns over qualitative data sharing and archiving. Challenges involved in anonymizing qualitative datasets were discussed. The chapter ended with an example of archiving qualitative data in one country, Poland. The next chapter centers on ethical issues involved with secondary qualitative data analysis.

References

Alderson, P. (1998). Confidentiality and consent in qualitative research. *Network-Newsletter of the British Sociological Association, 69*, 6–7.

Antes, A. L., Walsh, H. A., Strait, M., Hudson-Vitale, C. R., & Dubois, J. M. (2018). Examining data repository guidelines for qualitative data sharing. *Journal of Empirical Research on Human Research Ethics, 13*, 61–73.

Broom, A., Cheshire, L., & Emmison, M. (2009). Qualitative researchers' understandings of their practice and the implications for data archiving and sharing. *Sociology, 43*, 1163–1180.

Carlhed, C., & Alfredsson, I. (2009). Swedish National Data Service's strategy for sharing and mediating data: Practices of open access to and reuse of research data – The state of the art in Sweden 2009. 1 Assist's 35th Annual Conference, May 26–29, 2009, Tampere, Finland Retrieved from htts://mdh.diva-portal.org/smash/record.jsf?pid=diva2:279976

Cliggett, L. (2013). Qualitative data archiving in the digital age: Strategies for data preservation and sharing. *The Qualitative Report, 18*, 1–11.

DuBois, J. M., Strait, M., & Walsh, H. (2017). Is it time to share qualitative research data? *Qualitative Psychology*. Advance online publication. doi:10.1037/qup0000076

Elman, C., Kapiszewski, D., & Vinuela, L. (2010). Qualitative data archiving: Rewards and challenges. *Political Science and Politics, 43*, 23–27.

Kuula, A. (2011). Methodological and ethical dilemmas of archiving qualitative data. *IAssist Quarterly, 34*, 12–17.

Kuula, A., & Borg, S. (2008). Open access to and reuse a research data – the state of the art in Finland. *Finnish Social Science Data Archive, 7*. Retrieved from http://www.fsd. uta.fi/fi/ulkaisut/julkaisusarja/FSDjs07_OECD_en.pdf

Medjedović, I. (2011). Secondary analysis of qualitative interview data: Objections and experiences. Results of a German feasibility study. *Forum: Qualitative Social Research, 12*(3). Art. 10.

Niedbalski, J., & Ślezak, I. (2018). Ethical aspects of dissemination and archiving qualitative data in Poland. *Advances in Intelligent Systems and Computing, 621*, 181–259.

Richardson, J. C., & Godfrey, B. S. (2003). Towards ethical practice in the use of archived transcripted interviews. *Social Research Methodology, 6*, 347–355.

Roller, M. R., & Lavrakas, P. J. (2017). A total quality framework approach to sharing qualitative research data: Comment on Dubois et al. (2017). *Qualitative Psychology*. Advanced online publication. doi:10.1037/qup00000881

Saunders, B., Kitzinger, J., & Kitzinger, C. (2015). Anonymising interview data: Challenges and compromise in practice. *Qualitative Research, 15*, 616–632.

Travers, M. (2009). A not so strange silence: Why qualitative researchers should respond critically to the qualitative data archive. *Australian Journal of Social Issues, 44*, 273–289.

5

ETHICS IN SECONDARY QUALITATIVE DATA ANALYSIS

Secondary qualitative analysis raises ethical concerns regarding informed consent and confidentiality in reusing qualitative data which are addressed in this chapter along with perspectives from qualitative researchers and consumers on these issues. Best practices for anonymizing a qualitative text are identified along with standard protections of qualitative data in repositories. An example from one university's Institutional Review Board's (IRB's) guidance on secondary analysis of existing datasets is included, along with an example of informed consent from this author's phenomenological study on mothers, who have undergone traumatic birth experiences, interacting with their children. It provides permission for reuse of the interviews in the future by other researchers.

Researchers' and consumers' perspectives on ethical issues on reusing qualitative data

Yardley, Watts, Pearson, and Richardson (2014) conducted two discussion groups on ethical issues in reusing qualitative data. One group consisted of qualitative researchers and the second group of research consumers/users. Focus group data were analyzed for themes. Themes that emerged focused on the relationships forged between participants, interviewer, and academic institutions. Subthemes regarding these relationships included trust, sharing data, transparency and clarity, anonymity, permissions, and responsibility. Table 5.1 compares the perspectives of qualitative researchers and research participants on reusing qualitative data.

Informed consent

Bishop (2009) asked "Can consent for reuse be 'informed'?" (p. 262). The ethics of asking or of not asking for consent to reuse data is the focus here. Do qualitative

TABLE 5.1 Perspectives of researchers and research participants on reusing qualitative data

Relationships Subtheme	Examples from Research Participants	Examples from Researchers
Trust	Created by meeting researchers face to face and at institutional level.	Ethical and moral obligations distinguished.
	Participants made personal judgments about the researchers in primary studies before trusting them to utilize the data appropriately.	Concerns that repeated requests for consent to slight variations in data use or generalized consent forms could both create suspicion.
	Liked the idea of information about databases that demonstrated these were run by accredited academic institutions.	Uncertainty about how involved participants wanted to be in research beyond their initial participation.
Sharing data	Lack of understanding about the types of questions secondary analysis might be employed to answer and loss of richness/nuance in data.	Added layers of complexity for people unable to consent because of lack of capacity.
	Suggestion that better quality information is given by participants if they understand the purpose of the research.	Sometimes distance might be an advantage because the researcher's interpretation might be less affected by a sense of accountability to individual participants or their feelings about views expressed by participants.
	Important to understand the time frames and include data in reports but not a de facto reason not to use data.	Suggestion that systems and checks are needed to identify bona fide researchers with institutional support for their work.
	Societal changes also need to inform interpretations.	Concerns about protecting the reputation of the institution
Transparency and clarity	Dislike the term *reuse* because it was not easily understood, but did want a specific form of consent for any new research unrelated to original aims.	Need to balance the importance of following up interesting findings with the wishes of participants - a judgment that could depend on the ethical code a particular researcher ascribes to and his or her research questions.

Relationships Subtheme	Examples from Research Participants	Examples from Researchers
Anonymity, permissions, and responsibility	Anonymity considered vital to protect participants, but would also be interested if reuse of data resulted in new findings; how to achieve both was not resolved.	An individual or group of researchers reusing data they had collected to further explore unpredicted results considered a necessary activity for high-quality qualitative research.
	Concerns about group as well as individual identification.	It was suggested that the data be 'twice anonymized' to remove participant and researcher details before archiving in a centralized database.
	Expectation that data were already shared within research teams, and that when joining the team individuals would be briefed about expectations of data privacy.	Consent processes cannot be conducted as a "blanket" approach to cover every eventuality and still remain meaningful.
	Not the researcher's prerogative to restrict access to other bona fide researchers, but at the same time would not want carte blanche access.	Connections back to the original research team and/or participants might be useful but need mechanisms if they are untraceable.
		Some researchers believed they could act as proxy for participants in their study to make judgments on requests to reuse data in the specific instance of a new research proposal.

Reprinted with permission from Yardley et al. (2014) p. 107.

researchers have a moral responsibility to seek consent from their participants to reuse their data and/or to archive it? The relationship between qualitative researchers and their participants is very different that those of quantitative researchers. Bishop described the qualitative relationships as "infected in the data" (p. 296). This context of embeddedness of the data is a particular ethical challenge for secondary qualitative analysts. Participants in a qualitative study trust that the researcher will protect their data. Not knowing what use of the dataset in the future will entail, informed consent is obtained with general statements about how the data might be used. Bishop (2013) called for researchers in their ethical debates surrounding secondary qualitative analysis to engage moral theories and not just limit the discussion to concerns of particulars and situations.

Qualitative researchers are now beginning to address the issue of secondary analysis in their informed consent. There are three layers here regarding informed consent that qualitative researchers need to address (Alderson, 1998). The first involves the participants' informed consent for the original researcher to reuse the data. The second is for different researchers to have access to the participants' data to reanalyze it. The third involves the participants' consent, if the data are to be archived.

Preplanning for reuse of data with participants is best done during the initial consent process. The primary researcher can discuss with participants what may or may not be transcribed or recorded, etc. Conversations can be had around the option of data archiving, where data will be stored, and who will have access to the data. Once a qualitative dataset is available for secondary analysis, the primary researchers have no way of knowing in advance the specific research questions and research projects that secondary researchers will reuse the dataset for. So, how can the primary researchers when obtaining informed consent from their participants for reuse of their data make sure that the participants are truly "informed"? Corti, Van den Eynden, Bishop, and Wollard (2014) suggest that primary researchers provide some examples to the participants showing how similar datasets have been reused. Also, participants can be informed regarding possible options for limiting access to their data once their data are archived such as, restricting access to specific groups of users. Qualitative data archives have template permission forms that researchers can use.

As more and more funding agencies are requiring data sharing, permission must be made explicit in the initial informed consent. An example of guidance on secondary analysis of existing datasets from the IRB at the University of Connecticut (https://research.uconn.edu/irb/irb-forms-infoed) is located in Appendix A. Here is an excerpt from that university's IRB template for suggested statements for informed consent if researchers are interested in sharing their data:

> [If there is a possibility for future sharing of non-genetic research data/biological materials with other researchers or sharing of data per NIH & NSF data sharing requirements, insert one of the following two suggested statements, as appropriate, 1 – "[Data/biological materials] that we collect from you may be shared with other researchers in the future, linked together with other information such as your age, gender and ethnicity. We will share such information, but we will not give other researchers your name, address or phone number. There will be a code to link your [data/biological materials] with your name and other personal information." 2 – "[Data/biological materials] that we collect from you may be shared with other researchers in the future, but only after your name and all identifying information have been removed."]
>
> *(https://research.uconn.edu/irb/researcher-*
> *guidance/secondary-analysis-of-data-set/)*

An example of an informed consent that includes permission from the participants to have their data reused by other researchers is located in Appendix B;

the sentence giving this permission is bolded. This informed consent is modified from a phenomenological study that I have conducted on experiences of mothers who had traumatic births and their experiences interacting with their children.

Confidentiality

Confidentiality is another pertinent ethical issue in qualitative secondary analysis. Thorne (1998) brought up the element of non-maleficence regarding primary researchers' obligation to do no harm to their participants. Harm can be viewed as a violation of participants' privacy. A delicate balance is needed between researchers honoring their promise of confidentiality to their participants and at the same time retaining the usefulness of the data for future reuse by other researchers (Thomson, Bzdel, Golden-Biddle, Reay, & Estabrooks, 2005). Anonymization which involves de-identifying information of the participants from the dataset is one way to create a balance. The problem here, however, is that contextual information from specific, situation contexts that can be of value to secondary analysts is removed. If data are distorted to a degree, it lessens their potential value for reuse.

Prior to sharing a dataset with other researchers or before archiving it, anonymizing data is necessary to protect the participants' identities. A participant's identity can be disclosed from direct and indirect identifiers (Corti et al., 2014). Examples of direct identifiers include names, addresses, or telephone numbers. Indirect identifiers can include occupation, work place, or age.

Corti et al. (2014) have identified a list of best practices for anonymizing qualitative text: (p. 123)

- Do not collect disclosive data unless this is necessary, for example, do not ask for full names if they cannot be used;
- Plan anonymization at the time of transcription or initial write up, except for longitudinal studies where relationships between materials may require special attention during editing;
- Use pseudonyms or replacements that are consistent within the research team and throughout the project, for example, the same pseudonyms in publications or follow-up research;
- Use 'search and replace' techniques carefully, so the unintended changes are not made, and misspelled words are not missed;
- Identify replacements in text clearly: for example, with [brackets];
- Retain unedited versions of data for use within the research team and or preservation;
- Create an anonymization log of all replacements, aggregations or removals made, storing such a log separately from the anonymized data files.

In Table 5.2, Standard Protections of Qualitative Data repositories (Dubois, Strait, & Walsh 2017) are shown. These standards are listed for the repository, depositing researcher, and secondary data users. These protections are cumulative.

TABLE 5.2 Standard protections of qualitative data in repositories

Repository	Depositing Researcher	Secondary Data Users
Server is secured by firewalls and encryption.	Data must be de-identified, removing or changing as little as possible and as much as necessary.	Must not attempt to re-identify data that have been de-identified.
Depositing researchers must follow policies aimed at protecting participant information and scientific integrity.	For very sensitive data, entire cases may be removed.	Must securely store data.
Secondary data users must follow policies aimed at protecting participant information and scientific integrity.	*Or* If data are identifiable, REC approval and participant consent must be documented.	May not published identifiable information. May not redistribute data.
	For very sensitive de-identified data, this may also be required.	May not use for non-research or commercial purposes. Must cite original data source.

Note: Protections are cumulative across all three columns. Not all repositories have the same policies; these are sample elements of repository policies and practices. REC = Research Ethics Committee.

Reprinted with permission from DuBois et al. (2017, p. 7).

One example of additional protections necessary for sharing and archiving qualitative data

Hardy, Hughes, Hulen, and Schwartz (2016) warn that highly confidential and sensitive narratives from vulnerable populations participating in Community-Based Participatory Research (CBPR) required extra data management practices to protect the participants. Hardy et al. described the additional protections necessary to adhere to ethical standards while prioritizing data sharing regarding a CBPR with American Indians in Arizona regarding health resilience. A project-specific protocol was developed to strengthen trust between the researchers and project partners regarding concerns of data sharing and risks that may occur. In accordance with the Center for American Indian Resistance, subsets of de-identified data were made available to other researchers when those researchers made a formal request to use data for secondary analysis to the review team (Table 5.3).

In summary, ethical concerns regarding informed consent and confidentiality were covered in this chapter. Perspectives of both qualitative researchers

TABLE 5.3 Center for American Indian Resilience

Health Resilience Among American Indians in Arizona
Documenting and Promoting Resilience in Urban American Indians
Instructions for Access and use of Health Resilience Datasets

Introduction

In accordance with and in support of the Center for American Indian Resistance (CAIR), subset of de-identified data collected for pilot projects, *Health Resilience among American Indians in Arizona* (Northern Arizona University [NAU]) may be made available to collaborating researchers for valid research purposes wherein a formal request to make use of the data is submitted through the request process.

We have designed this plan to ensure protections and standards on data sharing and management in addition to each project's institutional review board (IRB) requirements. The maintenance of policies and standards of data management will ensure adherence to the goals of project research and a commitment to community engagement and trust between project partners and communities. Access to raw data will not be allowed unless investigators obtain permission from all project IRBs.

Section I. Application

To request access and permission to use/conduct secondary analysis data from *Health Resilience Among American Indians in Arizona* (NAU) a formal request must be submitted to the Review Team of the project including PIs (principle investigators) from Health Resilience, one PI from CAIR, and at least one project researcher from the core RARE team. This Review Team will use a set of questions to assess the adherence of the researcher request with the core principles of CAIR and Health Resilience.

Part A: Requestor information
1 Lead researcher's name, institution, email, and phone number
2 Researcher's relationship to CAIR and Health Resilience
3 Names of all other people working on the project including all co-investigators and research collaborators, including data analysts and research assistants. Each member of the project proposal is required to sign a Confidentiality Statement stating that they have read and will adhere to the conditions of the IRB. All members listed must submit proof of Responsible Conduct of Research (RCR) certification. The online training and certifications are available at no cost through the IRB offices at NAU.

Part B: Project information
1 Working title of potential project.
2 Brief description of the research project, including the research objectives or research question.
3 Data sets requested for the project including rationale for use of specific data sets.
4 Study design or methods and proposed analytical plan including time frame.
5 Budget and source of funds, if any.
6 Expected outputs (papers, graduate degree seeking research, conference papers, further grant applications, etc.)
7 Proposed order of authorship, and justification.

(Continued)

Section II. Use of research

Requests for access to data are considered by the project-specific Review Team.

If approved, the data are provided specifically for the analysis described in the application. Researchers will be required to submit brief annual reports to the Review Team from date of approval. Approval will be renewed following interim reports if work is progressing according to requestor's anticipated timeline and/or the timelines of CAIR (projects may not continue beyond funded period for CAIR).

Researchers must notify project Review Team with any substantial changes to the project by submitting a new application form and noting the amendment/s. Substantial changes include changes to the nature of the analysis, the topic addressed, or theoretical foundation (as it relates to the overarching goals of CAIR, CBPR, and community-engaged research); requests for additional variables or data sets; and the addition of any individual to the project. New collaborators are required to sign a Confidentially Statement prior to accessing any data.

Section III. Guidelines for public dissemination (publications and presentations)

Full acknowledgement of the source of data used must be provided in any publications or presentations that arise from access to, and use of, the data, included NIH project number, CAIR, and pilot project name and information.

Part A: Guidelines

- Researchers are required to follow their institutions' guides as well as IRB guidelines pertaining to publications and conference presentations.
- The preliminary authorship and order of authorship will be agreed upon with project PIs. Authors should ensure that research assistants, technical officers, and other 'non-authors' who contribute, including community members involved in supporting the project, are properly acknowledged. The acknowledgment may refer to any other persons who have provided comments, advice, support or other input into the paper, who are not already listed as authors. Permission should be sought from these persons before including their names.

Publications and journal submissions (including abstracts for conference presentations) must be reviewed and approved by the Review Team before submission to a journal or editor using the original application questions including the relationship between CAIR and Health Resilience goals and dissemination materials.

- In the event that a PI is not a co-author on a publication, authors must provide copies of publications to either or both of the PIs for *Health Resilience Among American Indians in Arizona and Documenting and Promoting Resilience in Arizona*

Part B: How to cite data

All publications that result from funding through CAIR must include the following acknowledgement:

Collection of the urban southern/northern Arizona American Indian data set was funded throughout the Center for American Indian Resilience, Northern Arizona University (5P20MD006872). Research reported in this publication was supported by the National Institute on Minority Health and Health Disparities of the National Institutes of Health under Award Number P20MD006872. The content is solely the responsibility of the authors and does not necessarily represent the official views of the National Institutes of Health.

Additional funding agencies should be acknowledged if this is applicable.

Reprinted with permission from Hardy et al. (2016) pp. 196–197.

and consumers regarding these ethical issues in qualitative secondary analysis were compared and contrasted. Examples were included from one university's IRB regarding guidance for secondary analysis of existing datasets, along with an example of informed consent that allows permission for reuse of the data by other researchers in the future. The next chapter centers on methodologies used in conducting reanalysis of qualitative datasets.

References

Alderson, P. (1998). Confidentiality and consent in qualitative research. *Network-Newsletter of the British Sociological Association, 69,* 6–7.

Bishop, L. (2009). Ethical sharing and reuse of qualitative data. *Australian Journal of Social Issues, 44,* 255–272.

Bishop, L. (2013). The value of moral theory for addressing ethical question when reusing qualitative data. *Methodological Innovations Online, 8,* 36–51.

Corti, L., Van den Eynden, V., Bishop, L., & Wollard, M. (2014). *Managing and sharing research data: A guide to good practice.* Los Angeles, CA: Sage.

DuBois, J. M., Strait, M., & Walsh, H. (2017). Is it time to share qualitative research data? *Qualitative Psychology.* doi:10.1037/gup0000076

Hardy, L. J., Hughes, A., Hulen, E., & Schwartz, A. L. (2016). Implementing qualitative data management plans to ensure ethical standards in multi-partner centers. *Journal of Empirical Research on Human Research Ethics, 11,* 191–198.

Thorne, S. (1998). Ethical and representational issues in qualitative secondary analysis. *Qualitative Health Research, 8,* 574–555.

Thomson, P., Bzdel, L., Golden-Biddle, K., Reay, T., & Estabrooks, C. A. (2005). Central questions of anonymization: A case study of secondary use of qualitative data. *Forum: Qualitative Social Research, 6*(1). Art. 29.

Yardley, S. J., Watts, K. M., Pearson, J., & Richardson, J. C. (2014). Ethical issues in the reuse of qualitative data: Perspectives from literature, practice, and participants. *Qualitative Health Research, 24,* 102–113.

6

PROCESS INVOLVED IN CONDUCTING A SECONDARY QUALITATIVE DATA ANALYSIS

Articles on the epistemological and ethical issues involved in secondary qualitative analysis and archiving have taken center stage over the years. There are far fewer publications focusing on the methodology involved in this type of analysis. Bright spots provided by Thorne (1994, 2013), Hinds, Vogel, and Clarke-Steffen (1997), and Heaton (2004) identified possible typologies of qualitative secondary analysis. In this chapter the process involved in conducting a secondary qualitative analysis is outlined. This chapter begins with a description of these typologies in the chronological order they were published in the literature. Examples of interdisciplinary studies are included to help illustrate these typologies. Armed with these typologies that secondary analysts can choose from, the remainder of the chapter focuses on the rest of the steps involved in conducting a secondary qualitative analysis starting with the research questions and ending with archiving the dataset. So many decisions need to be made as the secondary analyst travels along this process such as, which qualitative dataset to use, will the entire dataset or a subset be used, will supplementary data need to be collected, which typology to use, etc.

Thorne's typology

Thorne (1994) was the first person to develop a typology of secondary qualitative analysis. She identified five types: analytic expansion, retrospective interpretation, armchair induction, cross-validation, and amplified sampling (Table 6.1). Thorne (2013) noted that her typology of the five secondary data analysis approaches involves categories that are not mutually exclusive. Variations in design in each type are possible. Also, any of these types can be used as a part of an ongoing inquiry. Secondary data analysis can also lead to starting a new primary data collection.

TABLE 6.1 Thorne's approaches for secondary qualitative data analysis

Analytic expansion
In this approach, the secondary analyst uses the original dataset to ask a new question that had not been envisioned in the original study.

Retrospective interpretation
This is a type of analytic expansion which includes the temporal aspect of a research program which continues after the original findings had been published. Here the secondary analyst reuses the dataset to expand upon or develop further aspects that were only superficially addressed in the original dataset. Sometimes retrospective interpretation is done to correct findings that were the result of premature closure in the original study.

Armchair induction
Here, theoretical scholars who never entered the field reuse a dataset to produce findings different than those of primary researchers. These scholars reuse existing datasets with a perspectival distance from researchers who generated the data.

Cross-validation
In this approach the secondary analyst compares thematic conclusions from an original study across multiple datasets to confirm or to discount the original findings that the primary researcher may have missed. This provides a means to move beyond one specific sample and context to a more general claim.

Amplified sampling
This approach not only permits confirmability across distinct study contexts and populations but also for expansion of meaning by means of a wider lens.

Hinds, Vogel, and Clarke-Steffen's typology

Hinds et al. (1997) developed another typology of secondary qualitative data analysis. They defined secondary analysis as "The use of an existing dataset to find answers to a research question that differs from the question asked in the original or primary study" (p. 408). Four different types were identified.

1. In the secondary analysis the unit of analysis differs from that used in the primary study.
2. A subset of cases is chosen from the primary study to provide a more focused analysis.
3. The data from the primary study are reanalyzed to examine a concept that was not specifically addressed at that time. All or a portion of the original dataset can be reanalyzed.
4. Data from an existing qualitative study are used as one source of data while the researcher continues to define the study's methodology and collects additional data.

Heaton's typology

As illustrated in Table 6.2 Heaton (1998) first identified three types of secondary qualitative data analysis. First was an additional in-depth analysis which involves a more concentrated focus on a specific finding than was performed in the primary study. The second type involves an additional subset analysis where the researcher selects a subset of the sample from the primary study or studies for further analysis. Heaton called her third type a new perspective/conceptual focus. Here, retrospectively, a portion of a dataset or the entire dataset is analyzed using a different perspective to study concepts that were not the focus of the original research.

In 2004 Heaton developed a different typology that included five types of secondary qualitative analyses from an extensive review of secondary analysis studies published in the health and social care literature. Her typology was based on how secondary analysis was used in these research studies (Table 6.3). The first three types (supra analysis, supplementary analysis, and reanalysis) varied according to the degree to which the purposes of the original and secondary analysis converged or diverged. The last two types in Heaton's typology (amplified analysis and assorted analysis) are characterized by the number and nature of the datasets.

TABLE 6.2 Heaton's forms of secondary qualitative data analysis

	Nature of Original Data		
Main Focus of Analysis	*Single Qualitative Dataset*	*Multiple Qualitative Datasets*	*Mixed Qualitative and Quantitative Datasets*
Additional in-depth analysis	1a	1b	1c
Additional subset analysis	2a	2b	2c
New perspective/ conceptual focus	3a	3b	3c

Reprinted with permission from Heaton (1998).

TABLE 6.3 Heaton's types of secondary analysis of qualitative data

Supra analysis	Transcends the focus of the primary study from which the data were derived, examining new empirical, theoretical or methodological questions.
Supplementary analysis	A more in-depth investigation of an emergent issue or aspect of the data which was not considered or fully addressed in the primary study.
Reanalysis	Data are reanalyzed to verify and corroborate primary analyses of qualitative datasets.
Amplified analysis	Combines data from two or more primary studies for purposes of comparison or in order to enlarge a sample.
Assorted analysis	Combines secondary analysis of research data with primary research and/or analysis of naturalistic qualitative data.

Reprinted with permission from Heaton (2004, p. 38).

In her review of approximately 60 secondary qualitative analyses published in health and social care, Heaton (2004) used the following definition of secondary analysis to guide her selection of studies: "Secondary analysis is a research strategy which makes use of pre-existing quantitative data or pre-existing qualitative research data for the purposes of investigating new questions or verifying previous studies" (p. 16). After completing her review Heaton (2004) concluded that this definition did address the range of functions of secondary analysis for both types of data. It did not convey, however, the distinct features of qualitative secondary analysis. She identified four main characteristics of qualitative secondary analysis which were:

1. The focus of qualitative secondary analysis is on "non-naturalistic" data such as interviews.
2. Most of qualitative secondary analyses are based on the researchers' own previously collected data or through informal data sharing versus use of archival data.
3. Qualitative researchers develop particular approaches to secondary analysis, those being, the five types identified by Heaton.
4. Qualitative secondary analysis is perceived to be more problematic than quantitative secondary analysis.

Heaton's (2008) latest definition of secondary analysis of qualitative data is "the re-use of pre-existing qualitative data derived from previous research studies. These data include material such as semi-structured interviews, response to open ended questions in questionnaires, field notes and research diaries" (p. 34).

Interdisciplinary examples of Thorne's typology

The first two examples described here are from studies in my own program of research on traumatic childbirth. An example of Thorne's (1994, 2013) analytic expansion is provided by Puia, Lewis, and Beck (2013). The primary study was a mixed methods study on secondary traumatic stress in labor and delivery nurses (Beck & Gable, 2012). The secondary analysis only used the data from the qualitative strand where labor and delivery nurses described their experiences caring for women during traumatic births. In this secondary analysis Puia et al. focused on a subset of cases where nurses cared for families with a perinatal loss either due to an infant death or a fetal death. Three research questions guided this secondary analysis:

- What is the experience of nurses' caring for a patient during a fetal death?
- What is the experience of nurses' caring for a patient during an infant death?

- What are the similarities and differences in nurses' experiences in caring for a patient during a fetal death versus an infant death?

(Puia et al., 2013, p. 322)

Out of the 322 labor and delivery nurses who completed the qualitative strand of the original mixed methods study, 70 nurses described the experience of being present during a birth in which fetal death occurred. Another 85 nurses shared their experiences of caring for a patient during a birth in which an infant death happened. Krippendorff's (2013) content analysis revealed six overarching themes that emerged from both fetal and infant loss experiences: getting through the shift, symptoms of pain and loss, frustrations with inadequate care, showing genuine care, recovering from traumatic experience, and never forgetting.

In secondary qualitative reuse of data, content analysis can be used in different ways. Krippendorff's (2013) method for qualitative data can identify themes from the dataset or preset categories can be used for analysis. An example of using preset categories to reanalyze a qualitative dataset can be seen in Beck's (2018) secondary analysis of mistreatment of women during childbirth in healthcare facilities. Beck's (2004) phenomenological study of birth trauma was the original study. Thorne's (2013) analytic expansion was the secondary analysis type used. The new research question was "What are the categories of disrespect and abuse described in women's experiences of traumatic childbirth in high income countries?" (Beck, 2018, p. 97). The purpose of this secondary analysis was to identify the types and frequency of mistreatment of women during childbirth in high-income countries. Forty women participated in the original study. In this sample 23 mothers were from New Zealand, 8 from United States, 6 from Australia, and 3 from the United Kingdom. Bohren et al. (2015) developed a typology of mistreatment of women worldwide during childbirth in health-care facilities from a mixed-methods systematic review of research in low to middle income countries. Bohren and colleagues' typology provided the categories for the content analysis in this secondary analysis of mothers' descriptions of their traumatic births in high income countries. Seven categories are included in Bohren's typology: physical abuse, sexual abuse, verbal abuse, stigma and discrimination, failure to meet professional standards of care, poor rapport between women and providers, and health system conditions and constraints. Six of the seven categories of Bohren et al.'s (2015) typology were identified in Beck's (2018) secondary analysis. Sexual abuse was the only category not reported by women in high income countries. The top three categories of mistreatment revealed in this secondary analysis were failure to meet professional standards of care, poor rapport between women and providers, and verbal abuse.

Kelly, Pyke-Grimm, Stewart, and Hinds (2014) conducted a retrospective interpretation of two qualitative primary studies on childhood cancer treatment decision making of parents. The researchers examined these two grounded theory datasets to elaborate on one of the themes in the original studies, that being, parents' cancer communication, that was not fully investigated in the primary analysis. A subset of 23 of the 30 parents from the original sample was included in this secondary analysis. Included in this analysis were not only the interview transcripts but also field notes and theoretical memos. The new research question was "How do parents engage their ill children in cancer communication processes (information sharing and involvement of their children in treatment decision making)?" (Kelly et al., 2014, p. 514). This secondary analysis used Thorne's retrospective interpretation to elaborate on themes that were not fully analyzed in the primary studies. The secondary analysts did not have the original audiotapes to consult with because these had been destroyed after the original studies had been published as requested by the IRBs. Kelly et al. (2014) generated three hypotheses from their qualitative secondary analysis to guide their future research:

> Hypothesis 1: Parents, their children, and clinicians take different actions regarding information sharing and treatment decision making that might be discordant, complementary, or in agreement.
>
> Hypothesis 2: Parents described sharing information with and involving their children in treatment decision making at the same time in multiple interviews; how these two cancer communication strategies are linked needs to be defined.
>
> Hypothesis 3: There are varying patterns of family treatment decision making that can be described by how information is shared with the child and the child's involvement in treatment decision making.
>
> *(p. 529)*

In Kelly and colleagues' secondary analysis, two of the three secondary analysts had been involved in the two original studies and were able to provide valuable contextual understanding to the relationships among persons in the interviews. Kelly et al. warned that secondary qualitative analysts have a challenge not to exaggerate the primary studies' findings as a result of incomplete contextual understanding. To avoid overrepresentation of some parents' experiences which could lead to bias, Kelly and colleagues did not draw conclusions based on the frequency of parents' comments in the primary studies.

Interdisciplinary examples of Hinds, Vogel, and Clarke-Steffen's typology

An illustration of Hinds et al.'s (1997) second type of qualitative secondary analysis, extracting subsets of cases for a similar but more focused analysis, is my (Beck, 2013) secondary analysis of the obstetric nightmare of shoulder dystocia (Figure 6.1). Here, two datasets from two different samples were reanalyzed to increase the generalization of the findings. The first original study was a phenomenological study of 23 mothers' experiences of children with obstetric brachial plexus injuries due to shoulder dystocia (Beck, 2009). The second primary study

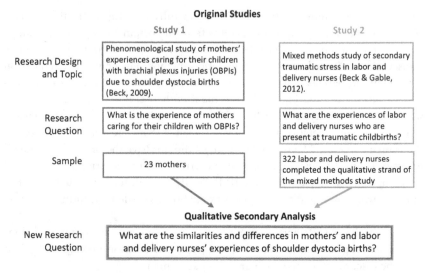

FIGURE 6.1 Secondary analysis of the obstetric nightmare of shoulder dystocia.

was the qualitative strand of a mixed methods study of secondary traumatic stress in labor and delivery nurses (Beck & Gable, 2012). This secondary analysis compared traumatic experiences of shoulder dystocia from the mothers' and nurses' perspectives. Subsets from each of the two studies were used for this secondary analysis. In Beck's (2009) phenomenological study, only the data from mothers who described in-depth their shoulder dystocia births were included. In the mixed methods study (Beck & Gable, 2012) only data from the qualitative strand where nurses had described shoulder dystocia as the traumatic birth they had attended were selected for inclusion. In this secondary analysis I used Krippendorff's (2013) content analysis to identify themes. Comparing and contrasting the two datasets of different perspectives of shoulder dystocia births revealed four themes: in the midst of the obstetric nightmare, reeling from the trauma that just transpired, enduring heartbreak: the heavy toll on mothers, and haunted by memories: the heavy toll on nurses. This secondary analysis revealed striking similarities on how mothers and nurses perceived this obstetric nightmare.

Citing Hinds et al.'s (1997) typology, Bernhofer and Sorrell (2015) extracted a subset of cases and analyzed these to provide answers to new research questions that provided a more focused analysis. Bernhofer and Sorrell's original study was a grounded theory of 48 nurses' decisions when caring for hospitalized patients with chronic and acute pain. One of the four core concepts that emerged in the primary data was moral distress. The purpose of their secondary analysis study was to focus further on nurses' experiences of moral distress when they felt constrained in caring for their patients with optimal pain management. Members of the primary research team conducted this analysis. The analysts listened to all 48 original audio recordings plus reviewed all interview transcripts and written notes. Findings highlighted the frustration nurses experienced due to being unable to manage their patients' pain. Barriers to managing patients' pain focused on the nurses' difficulty communicating with or obtaining necessary orders from physicians and a lack of pain management education.

Interdisciplinary examples of Heaton's typology

Coming from the discipline of social work is an example of Heaton's (2004) supra analysis. In the United States, Maguire-Jack and Negash (2015) conducted a secondary qualitative analysis of barriers in access to child maltreatment prevention programs for families involved with child protective services. The original study investigated the impact of maltreatment prevention programs on child protective services workers' decision making (Maguire-Jack & Byers, 2014). Semi-structured interviews with open-ended questions were conducted with 13 child protective services workers and supervisors. The purpose of the primary study was to examine child protective services workers' use of their knowledge of maltreatment prevention programs on how they decided whether or not to screen cases for maltreatment allegations and to remove children from their homes and place them into substitute care. The primary researchers noticed that there was a divergence between the data collected by means of their semi-structured questions and the open-ended questions. So, in their supra analysis, Maguire-Jack and Negash (2015) examined a new empirical question, focusing specifically on the barriers that child protective workers faced with child maltreatment prevention programs. Two overarching themes were found. One theme related to barriers families in child protective services faced when accessing prevention programs. The second theme focused on barriers that prevented child protective services workers from making referrals to prevention programs.

In Australia researchers conducted an example of Heaton's (2004) supplementary analysis (Jose et al., 2017). The lead author is a physiotherapist and this qualitative secondary analysis focused on the understanding of gender influences on the processes leading up to weight loss surgery. This secondary analysis came from a larger study exploring weight loss patients' expectations and experiences via focus groups. Discussion in the focus groups centered on reasons for the decision to have weight loss surgery, experiences and expectations of surgery, and information and support provided. Participants were also asked to discuss gender differences. This secondary analysis provided a more in-depth examination of gender differences regarding weight loss surgery which had not been completely addressed in the primary study. Focus group transcripts from 49 participants were reanalyzed with the lens now focused on gender differences. Secondary analysis revealed the biggest differences in women and men related to mechanisms underlying weight gain, living in a big body, differences in social and cultural expectations having to do with their disclosure to have surgery, interactions with clinicians, and sense of self after surgery.

Heaton's (2004) amplified analysis type of qualitative secondary data analysis was used by researchers in the United Kingdom to examine patients' priorities in osteoarthritis and comorbid conditions (Cheraghi-Sohi et al., 2013). In their secondary analysis datasets from four different qualitative studies were combined to explore new research questions. A total of 30 participants with osteoarthritis and comorbidities from the four studies comprised the sample for the secondary analysis. Foci of these four studies concentrated on the experiences and beliefs of persons with knee osteoarthritis. The purpose of this secondary analysis was to investigate how patients prioritize osteoarthritis among their comorbidities and whether these priorities change over time. Analysis revealed three groups of participants. The first group consistently identified osteoarthritis as their main condition; the second group did not identify osteoarthritis as their main condition, and third was the group where the priority of their main conditions changed over time.

Assorted analysis is Heaton's (2004) fourth type of qualitative secondary analysis. Redman-MacLaren, Mills, and Tommbe (2014) in Australia combined existing qualitative data from a prior original study with new data from an ongoing study. Using interpretive focus groups with women in Papua New Guinea the lead researcher, who is a social worker, and her team extended their analysis of existing qualitative data with new data to inform their grounded theory study on how women experience male circumcision. The grounded theory study used existing data from a large mixed methods study of male circumcision. The first author was the project manager for that study involving 64 women and led many of the focus groups. New data were collected in two steps. First, participants were invited to interpret parts of their data, "data chunks," from the original study. The second step involved storyboarding, which used visual arts for participatory research. Participants drew storyboards of their interpretations of their "data chunks." Use of constant comparative method in this secondary analysis supplemented with new data led to a tentative transformational grounded theory.

Heaton's (2004) supra analysis approach was used in a secondary analysis of the challenge to health professionals when carers resist truth telling at the end of life (Nobel, Price, & Porter, 2014). Two primary studies in the United Kingdom, which investigated staff's perspectives in a palliative children's setting and in a palliative adult setting using focus groups, were reanalyzed to examine new theoretical questions focusing on common issues in each primary study. Secondary analysis revealed that both the adult and pediatric palliative care staff were caught in a dilemma, subject to policies that promoted openness in planning for their patients' deaths and to family caregivers who many times prevented them from being truthful with their patients about their upcoming death.

In Canada, five qualitative studies' findings were combined in a secondary qualitative data analysis using Heaton's amplified analysis. Men's health seeking behavior regarding bone health following a fragility fracture was the topic (Sale, Ashe, Beaton, Bogosch, & Frankel, 2016). All five of the original studies were phenomenological studies. Sale was the first author in all the five published studies coming from the Institute of Health Policy, Management & Evaluation at the University of Toronto. In each of the five primary studies, both men and women were recruited, but the number of men enrolled in the studies only ranged from two to seven. Sale and colleagues decided to combine the existing qualitative datasets so there would be enough data to focus specifically on the experiences and behavior of men. A total of 22 males comprised this secondary analysis sample. Results revealed that few of the men had added any behaviors at all to their daily routine regarding bone health recommendations. Some of the men admitted to risk-taking practices in relation to their bone health. Wives and other women in their lives played a significant role in their bone health behavior. Last, men did not express concern about their bone health.

Research process involved in secondary qualitative analysis

Figure 6.2 displays the process required from start to finish in a secondary qualitative data analysis. With any research study what drives the methodology are

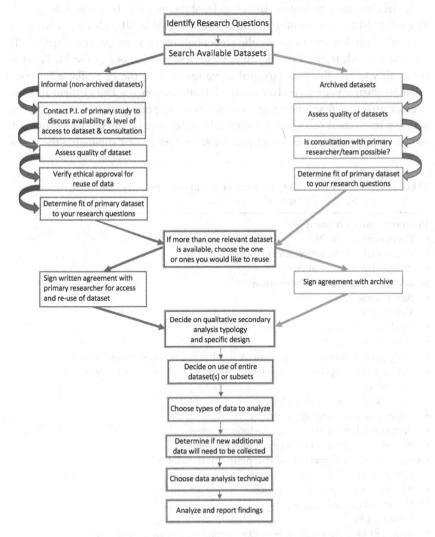

FIGURE 6.2 Steps of research process involved in secondary qualitative analysis.

the research questions that are to be answered. Secondary qualitative analysis is no different. Research questions will guide the secondary analyst's decision of which qualitative dataset to choose. Is there an appropriate match between the research questions and the dataset being considered? Unless researchers are going to reuse their own qualitative dataset, the search for one to use can be time-consuming. Will the researcher search through available archived datasets? Or will the researcher consider asking colleagues, who have relevant qualitative datasets, if they are willing to share their datasets? With the upswing in mixed methods studies, secondary analysts should not only search qualitative datasets but also mixed methods ones. The qualitative strand in a mixed methods study can provide a rich data source for reuse.

In deciding on a qualitative dataset, its feasibility needs to be assessed along with its quality. Many criteria go into this assessment (Table 6.4). This starts with the original research team. What are the credentials of the Principal Investigator (PI) and the research team? Take the time to review publications of the PI. What is the quality of the PI's previous qualitative research? Is the PI available for consultation during your secondary analysis? Consultation is a key element in your decision making. A secondary analyst may need to periodically consult with the primary researchers to answer questions about context and methodology used. A signed agreement between the PI and the secondary analyst stipulating the terms

TABLE 6.4 Criteria for deciding whether or not to use a primary qualitative dataset for the feasibility of secondary analysis

Primary research team
- Credentials of the PI
- Credentials of the entire research team
- Availability for consultation

Available contextual information
- Audiotapes
- Videotapes
- Field notes/memos
- Whole interviews
- Only parts of interviews (need discursive history of interviewers' responses)
- Detailed transcription of interviews (interaction between interviewer and interviewee)
- How interviewers were selected
- Time, place, and setting of interviews
- Background characteristics of the interviewers
- Background characteristics of the interviewees

Completeness and quality of the primary dataset
- Complete data for every participant
- Richness and depth of interviews
- Quality of the audiotapes
- Missing data
- Sufficient data are available to answer secondary research questions

of agreement should be executed. If using an archived dataset, there is also a signed agreement that will be required.

Important information on just how much of the original dataset the secondary analyst will be privy to needs to be assessed. Will only transcripts of the interviews be available? Or will audiotapes or videotapes of the interviews also be a part of the accessible dataset? Field notes and memos are excellent additions to an accessible dataset as they help add valuable context of the primary study. How detailed are the transcripts of the interviews? Is the interaction between the interviewers and the participants part of the transcripts? Does the dataset include the time, place, and setting of the interviews? What are the background characteristics of both the interviewers and the participants? How rich and in-depth are the interviews? Are the interviews only on a superficial level? If audiotapes are available, what is their quality? Also, you need to verify that ethical approval for reuse of the dataset was received. All these questions will help in the decision of the fit of a particular primary dataset with a secondary analyst's research questions. There is a possibility that more than one primary dataset may be needed to answer the research questions. Another major decision concerns which secondary qualitative analysis typology to use.

One has to also consider the secondary analysts' relationship to the original dataset (Table 6.5). One relationship occurs when the original researchers are conducting a reuse of their own dataset. In this case the options include the original researchers reanalyzing one primary dataset or multiple ones. The original researchers may also choose to add new authors and/or new supplementary data. The option is also available for original researchers to combine their dataset with other primary researchers' datasets. The second relationship occurs when secondary analysts, who

TABLE 6.5 Secondary analyst's relationship to primary research

Original researcher
- Original researcher(s) reanalyze one primary dataset
- Original researcher(s) reanalyze multiple datasets
- Original researcher(s) reanalyze primary dataset(s) with new author(s)
- Original researcher(s) reanalyze primary dataset(s) plus collect new supplementary data
- Original researcher(s) reanalyze dataset with new additional authors plus collect new supplementary data
- Multiple original researchers combine their datasets and reanalyze them together
- Multiple original researchers combine their datasets and reanalyze with new additional authors

Secondary analyst
- Secondary analyst(s) with no previous involvement collaborate with original researcher(s)
- Secondary analyst(s) with no previous involvement alone with original dataset
- Secondary analyst(s) with prior involvement with original dataset collaborating with original researcher(s)
- Secondary analyst(s) with prior involvement with original dataset not collaborating with original researcher(s)

were not the PIs of the original study, want to reuse a primary dataset. Was the secondary analyst involved in some way with the primary study or not? Will the secondary analyst collaborate with the original researchers or not?

Sample is yet another consideration. Will the secondary analyst use an entire dataset(s) or subset(s)? Will there be a need to collect new supplementary data to fully answer the research questions? The next decision involves how the data will be analyzed. Popular options include content analysis, thematic analysis, constant comparative analysis, phenomenological analysis, and metaphor analysis. What does the secondary analyst foresee as the outcome of the analysis: themes, categories, concepts, models, narratives, grounded theory, interpretive description, or metaphors, to name a few.

In summary, three different typologies of secondary qualitative analyses were described in this chapter: Thorne's, Hinds et al.'s, and Heaton's. Examples of secondary qualitative analyses conducted by researchers from various disciplines were presented to illustrate use of these typologies. The second part of the chapter focused on the steps involved in conducting a secondary qualitative analysis. Qualitative data archives are explored in Chapter 7.

References

Beck, C. T. (2004). Birth trauma: In the eye of the beholder. *Nursing Research, 53,* 28–35.

Beck, C. T. (2009). The arm: There is no escaping the reality for mothers of children with obstetric brachial plexus injuries. *Nursing Research, 58,* 237–245.

Beck, C. T. (2013). The obstetric nightmare of shoulder dystocia: A tale from two perspectives. *MCN: American Journal of Maternal Child Nursing, 38,* 34–40.

Beck, C. T. (2018). A secondary analysis of mistreatment of women during childbirth in health care facilities. *Journal of Obstetric, Gynecologic, and Neonatal Nursing, 47,* 94–104.

Beck, C. T., & Gable, R. K. (2012). A mixed methods study: Secondary traumatic stress in labor and delivery nurses. *Journal of Obstetric, Gynecologic, and Neonatal Nursing, 41,* 747–760.

Bernhofer, E. I., & Sorrell, J. M. (2015). Nurses managing patients' pain may experience moral distress. *Clinical Nursing Research, 24,* 401–414.

Bohren, M. A., Vogel, J. P., Hunter, E. C., Lutsiv, O., Makh, S. K., Souza, J. P., ... Gulmezoglu, M. (2015). The mistreatment of women during childbirth in health care facilities globally: A mixed-methods systematic review. *PLOS Medicine, 12*(6). E1001847. doi:10.1371/journal.pmed.10001847

Cheraghi-Sohi, S., Bower, P., Kennedy, A., Morden, A., Rogers, A., Richardson, J., ... Ong, B. N. (2013). Patient priorities in osteoarthritis and comorbid conditions: A secondary analysis of qualitative data. *Arthritis Care & Research, 65,* 920–927.

Heaton, J. (1998, October). Secondary analysis of qualitative data. *Social Research Update,* Issue 22, University of Surrey.

Heaton, J. (2004). *Reworking qualitative data.* Thousand Oaks, CA: Sage.

Heaton, J. (2008). Secondary analysis of qualitative data: An overview. *Historical Social Research, 33,* 33–45.

Hinds, P. S., Vogel, R. J., & Clarke-Steffen, L. (1997). The possibilities and pitfalls of doing a secondary analysis of a qualitative data set. *Qualitative Health Research, 7,* 408–424.

Jose, K., Venn, A., Sharman, M., Wilkinson, S., Williams, D., & Ezzy, D. (2017). Understanding the gendered nature of weight loss surgery: Insights from an Australian Qualitative study. *Health Sociology Review, 26,* 113–127.

Kelly, K. P., Pyke-Grimm, K., Stewart, J. L., & Hinds, P. S. (2014). Hypothesis generation for childhood cancer communication research: Results of secondary analysis. *Western Journal of Nursing Research, 36,* 512–533.

Krippendorff, K. (2013). *Content analysis: An introduction to its methodology.* Thousand Oaks, CA: Sage.

Maguire-Jack, K., & Byers, K. (2014). The impact of prevention programs on decisions in child protective services. *Child Welfare, 92,* 59–86.

Maguire-Jack, K., & Negash, T. (2015). Barriers in access to child maltreatment prevention programs for families involved with child protective services. *Journal of Child Custody, 12,* 152–174.

Nobel, H., Price, J. E., & Porter, S. (2014). The challenge to health professionals when carers resist truth telling at the end of life: A qualitative secondary analysis, *Journal of Clinical Nursing, 24,* 927–936.

Puia, D. M., Lewis, L., & Beck, C. T. (2013). Experiences of obstetric nurses who are present of a perinatal loss. *Journal of Obstetric, Gynecologic, and Neonatal Nursing, 42,* 321–331.

Redman-MacLaren, M., Mills, J., & Tommbe, R. (2014). Interpretive focus groups: A participatory method for interpreting and extending secondary analysis of qualitative data. *Global Health Action, 7,* 25214. doi:10.3402/qhav7.25214

Sale, J. E., Ashe, M. C., Bogoch, E., & Frankel, L. (2016). Men's health seeking behaviours regarding bone health after a fragility fracture: A secondary analysis of qualitative data. *Osteoporosis International, 10,* 3113–3119.

Thorne, S. (1994). Secondary analysis in qualitative research: Issues and implications. In J. M. Morse (Ed.), *Critical issues in qualitative research methods* (pp. 263–279). Thousand Oaks, CA: Sage.

Thorne, S. (2013). Secondary qualitative data analysis. In C. T. Beck (Ed.), *Routledge international handbook of qualitative nursing research* (pp. 393–416). New York: Routledge.

7

INTERNATIONAL QUALITATIVE DATA ARCHIVES

This chapter begins with the research data life cycle which extends the research process beyond just disseminating research findings. It addresses archiving qualitative data so data are preserved for reuse by other researchers. Qualitative data archives in the United Kingdom, United States, Europe, and Australia are described. Qualitative data repository guidelines are also included in this chapter.

Research data life cycle

As data sharing and secondary qualitative data analysis gain popularity, the typical research cycle needs to be extended. No longer is a research project considered complete when its findings have been disseminated. Use of the concept of the research data life cycle extends this to digital preservation and data curation practices (Corti, Van den Eynden, Bishop, & Woollard, 2014). The steps in the research data life cycle are listed in Table 7.1. Steps toward the end of the cycle bring new extended life to a dataset through preservation and reusing the data in secondary qualitative data analysis. The Data Documentation Initiative (DDI) was developed in 1995 as a standard for social science data with the idea of the extended data life cycle (DDI Alliance, 2017). Figure 7.1 provides an illustration of the phases in the DDI life cycle as diagrammed by the Inter-university Consortium for Political and Social Research (ICPSR) which resides at the University of Michigan (https://www.icpsr.umich.edu).

To help with the concern of the secondary analyst "not having been there," metadata, which is data about data, can be created. Though a time-consuming activity for the primary researchers, the benefits of a high quality metadata for secondary analysts are many and valuable. The DDI (www.ddialliance.org) is an international standard that can be used to create a metadata for both quantitative and qualitative research in social science. In addition to the name of the Principal

TABLE 7.1 Typical activities undertaken in the research data life cycle

Activity	Key Features
Discovery and planning	Designing research
	Planning data management
	Planning consent for sharing
	Planning data collection, processing protocols and templates
	Finding and discovering data sources
Data collection	Collecting data-recording, observation, measurement, experimentation and simulation
	Capturing and creating metadata
	Acquiring existing third-party data
Data processing and analysis	Entering data, digitizing, transcribing, and translation
	Checking, validating, cleaning, and anonymizing data where necessary
	Deriving data
	Describing and documenting data
	Analyzing data
	Interpreting data
	Producing research outputs
	Authoring publications
	Citing data sources
	Managing and storing data
Publishing and sharing	Establishing copyright of data
	Creating discovery metadata and user documentation
	Publishing or sharing data
	Distributing data
	Controlling access to data
	Promoting data
Long-term management	Migrating data to best format
	Migrating data to suitable medium
	Backing up and storing data
	Gathering and producing metadata and documentation
	Preserving and curating data
Reusing data	Conducting secondary analysis
	Undertaking follow-up research
	Conducting research reviews
	Scrutinizing findings
	Using data for teaching and learning

Reprinted with permission from Corti et al. (2014, pp. 17–18).

Investigator (PI), title of the study, and description of the project, some of the other key metadata elements identified by the DDI include funding sources, data collectors, sample description, data sources, unit of analysis, variables, instruments used to collect data, interview guide, coding instruments, and any related publications.

In metadata for a qualitative dataset field notes can be valuable in documenting contextual information. With the increasing use of data sharing, Phillippi and

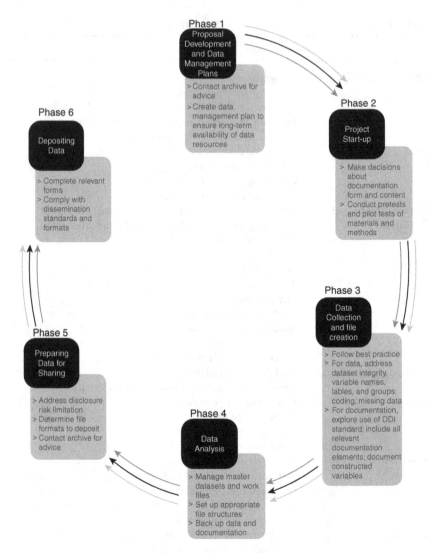

FIGURE 7.1   Phases of the research data life cycle (https://www.icpsr.umich.edu).

Lauderdale (2018) developed a guide to field notes to help provide rich context beyond the original research team. Figure 7.2 is a guide for individual interviews or focus groups, while Figure 7.3 is a guideline for the context of a full study. Phillippi and Lauderdale emphasized the fluid nature of field notes in qualitative research and that researchers are encouraged to modify the content based on their methodology. For field notes about the study context, the authors included five major components: basic information, geographic setting, demographics, societal pressures, and cost of living. For field notes about interviews or focus groups the major components include the setting, participants, the interview, and critical reflection.

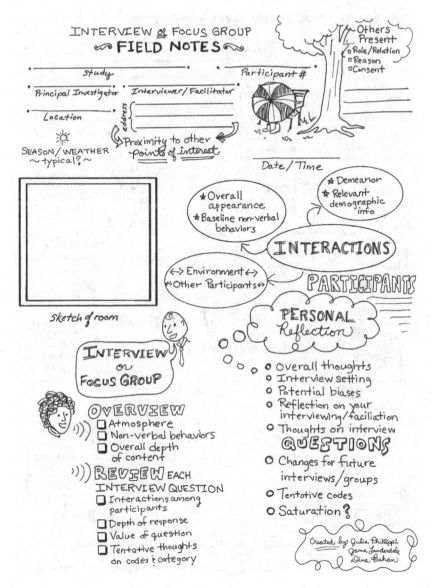

FIGURE 7.2 Interview or focus group field notes.
Reprinted with permission from Phillippi and Lauderdale (2018) Supplemental material.

Developments in providing secure access to disclosed data occurred in 2008 in the United States and 2011 in the United Kingdom. In the United States the National Opinions Research Center started the first "Data Enclave," which provided a protected virtual environment where researchers, who were authorized, could access sensitive data (Lana, Heus, & Mulcahy, 2008). Next, in 2011, in the United Kingdom, a Secure Data Service (SDS)

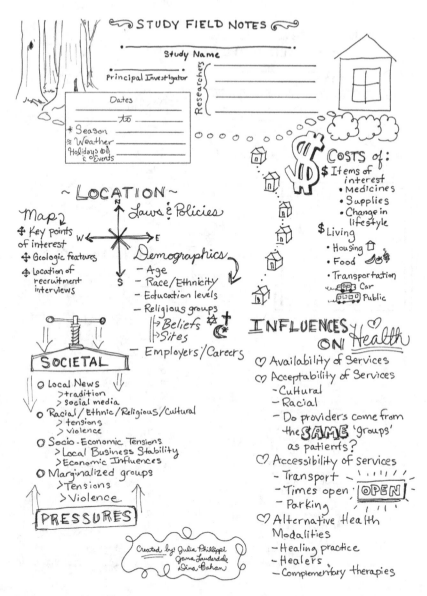

FIGURE 7.3 Field notes about study context.
Reprinted with permission from Phillippi and Lauderdale (2018) Supplemental material.

was set up for researchers to access remotely business, economic, and social data which were considered too specific, confidential, and sensitive to be made available under regular licenses of regular data services (SDS, 2011). Also during this time period, universities had taken on more responsibility to support their researchers, staff, and their datasets and to develop institutional repositories.

Qualitative data archives

United Kingdom qualitative archives

U.K. Data Service

U.K. Data Service provides the United Kingdom's largest collection of U.K. and international social, economic, and population data. It is funded by the Economic and Social Research Council (ESRC). The U.K. Data Service collection includes qualitative data. The qualitative database began as Qualidata in 1994. Qualidata was housed within the Department of Sociology at the University of Essex (the ESRC Qualitative Data Archival Resource Center). The purpose of Qualidata was not to serve as an archive but to act as the middleman between qualitative researchers and existing archives. Qualidata's role was to locate, evaluate, process, and catalogue the qualitative data. Next it arranged for the deposit of that qualitative dataset to an appropriate archive.

In 1995, the ESRC Datasets Policy was established. A condition of ESRC research funding was depositories of machine and non-machine qualitative data within three months of the end of the award. Spearheading the efforts of U.K. Data Service is Louise Corti who was its Associate Director. In 2003, Qualidata became part of the ESDS. In 2012 it became a fully integrated into the U.K. Data Service.

The Timescapes Archive

The Timescapes Archive specializes in qualitative longitudinal data which forms part of an institutional repository at the University of Leeds and conforms to international archiving standards (OAIS). It was developed in 2007–2012 under the ESRC Timescapes Initiative for Qualitative Longitudinal Research (www. timescapes.leeds.ac.uk). This archive was designed as a complementary resource to the U.K. Data Archive (it opened to users in mid-2010). It is able to archive data from the public section of non-ESRC funded studies. Primary researchers from five universities (Leeds, London South Bank, Open University, Cardifford, and Edinburgh) collaborated working from a variety of disciplines (sociology, social psychology, social policy, oral history, health studies, and cultural studies) to develop Timescapes (Neale, Henwood, & Holland, 2012). Their individual projects investigated siblings and friendships in childhood, lives of teenagers, motherhood, men as fathers, work-life balance in families who were raising young children, grandparents and the oldest generation. All together these longitudinal qualitative research projects have followed the lives of more than 300 individuals. The primary researchers are encouraged to reuse their own data and link them to their current research as it progresses. Primary and secondary qualitative analysis are thereby combined to increase the use of their evidence.

In Timescapes retrospective life history data are included to put data that are prospectively collected to follow the participants' lives as they unfold. This resource contains data from eight core Timescapes projects that span the life course (Neale & Bishop, 2012). The datasets are interlinked providing the ability to track individual and families over time examining personal relationship and identities. Secondary analysts can search these datasets for thematic content using key words.

A template from Timescapes Archive for informed consent can be found in Table 7.2. Data in the Timescapes Archive has four levels of access:

TABLE 7.2 Timescapes Archive consent form template

timescapes

An ESRC Qualitative Longitudinal Study

Consent Form for [name of project]

Please tick the appropriate boxes

I have read and understood the project information sheet dated DD/MM/YYYY. ☐
I have been given the opportunity to ask questions about the project. ☐
I agree to take part in the project. Taking part in the project will include being interviewed ☐
and recorded (audio or video). [Other forms of participation can be listed].
I understand that my taking part is voluntary; I can withdraw from the study at any ☐
time and I will not be asked any questions about why I no longer want to take part.
Select only one of the next two options:

I would like my name used where what I have said or written as part of this study ☐
will be used in research reports and any other publications so that anything I have
contributed to this project can be recognised.
I do not want my name used in this project. ☐
I understand my personal details such as phone number and address will not be ☐
revealed to people outside the project.
I understand that my words may be quoted in publications, reports, web pages, and ☐
other research outputs but my name will not be used unless I requested it above.
I agree for my data to be archived at a facility operated by the University of Leeds and ☐
the UK Data Archive at the University of Essex. [More detail can be provided here
so that decisions can be made separately about audio, video, etc.]
I understand that other researchers will have access to this data only if they agree ☐
to preserve the confidentiality of that data and if they agree to the terms I have
specified in this form.
I understand that other researchers may use my words in publications, reports, web pages, ☐
and other research outputs according to the terms I have specified in this form.
I agree to assign the copyright I hold in any materials related to this project to [name of ☐
researcher].

_____   _____   _____
Name of Participant   Signature   Date

_____   _____   _____
Researcher   Signature   Date

Contact details for further information: Names, phone, email addresses, etc.

(www.timescapes.leeds.ac.uk)

1. Public access
2. Registered access to anonymized data that are available to researchers who have professional credentials
3. Restricted access to data that are sensitive or difficult to anonymize. Researchers need to apply and receive approval from the originating team
4. Closed access to embargoed data (Neale, 2013).

The United States qualitative archives

Inter-university Consortium for Political and Social Research (ICPSR)

The ICPSR resides in the Institute for Social Research at the University of Michigan (http://www.isr.umich.edu). It was established in 1962 for quantitative data and began archiving qualitative data since 2011. The consortium has approximately 759 universities, government agencies, and other institutions. Member institutions' faculty, students, and staff have full and direct access to the data archive. The ICPSR also provides training and instructional resources to help users of the archived data. The consortium has archived more than 250,000 files of research in the field of social and behavioral sciences.

Qualitative Data Repository

The Qualitative Data Repository's (QDR) mission is to archive for storing and sharing digital data and its related documentation for qualitative and multi-method research in the social sciences. The National Science Foundation funds QDR and the archive is hosted by Syracuse University in their Center for Qualitative and Multi-Method Inquiry. Political science is the initial emphasis of QDR. Researchers can deposit digital data in a variety of formats—alphanumeric, audio, video, and photographic. The staff at QDR can scan data that researchers have only in hard copy form.

In QDR, three types of data projects are distinguished: active citation compilations, data collections, and topic clusters (Elman & Kapiszewski, 2013). The first type, active citation, increases transparency for researchers to show and allow readers to see the evidence that the researchers relied on. Data sources and claims are supported by annotated citations hyperlinked to the sources themselves (Moravcsik, 2010). Readers can evaluate the claim made by researchers in published scholarship. The second type of data projects are data collections which are used for secondary analysis. Topic clusters are the third type and can be used by scholars to learn relevant background information as they develop their research projects.

Henry A. Murray Research Archive

The Murray Research Archive was founded at the Radcliffe College at Harvard University in 1976. It is an endowed repository at Harvard University for qualitative and quantitative research data. In 2005 the archive joined with the Institute for Quantitative Social Sciences. Emphasis is on longitudinal studies on human development and social change, with special focus on the lives of American women. The Murray Center not only is a repository for longitudinal data but also provides training for researchers in the use of existing datasets. To ensure long-term continual access to digital data, a systematic data migration plan was designed. The Murray Research Archive will move data from any storage media, data format, or related hardware or software that is becoming obsolete to a new updated media, format, hardware and/or software.

National Institute of Health (NIH)

The National Institute of Health (NIH) has a data sharing policy. The NIH "expects investigators seeking more than $500K in direct support in any given year to submit a data sharing plan with their application or to indicate why data sharing is not possible" (http://www.nlm.nih.gov/hihbmic/nih_data_sharing_policies.html). In preparing a data sharing plan under NIH extramural support, the NIH identified the following key elements to include:

- What data will be shared?
- Who will have access to the data?
- Where will the data to be shared be located?
- When will the data be shared?
- How will researchers locate and access the data? (http://sharing.nih.gov)

European qualitative archives

A list of these archives was obtained from the U.K. Data Service website (www.ukdataservice.ac.uk). Many of these archives are part of the council of European Social Science Data Archives (CESSDA).

Austria

The Austrian Ministry of Science and Research supports the Wiener Institute for Social Science Data Documentation and Methods (Wisdom). It was founded in 1985 and in 2007 it extended its scope to acquired qualitative and mixed method datasets (Smioski, 2010/2011).

Czech Republic

The Czech Sociological Data Archive (SDA) collaborates with the Institute of Sociology of the Academy of Sciences of the Czech Republic to archive qualitative data (Cízek, 2010/2011).

Finland

The Finnish Social Science Data Archive (FSD) has collected and archived qualitative collections since 1999. All the quantitative and qualitative datasets that are archived at the FSD have an overview of the dataset and the methodology in English. FSD will translate qualitative data (questions and response categories) on request free of charge. FSD does not provide translation of the qualitative datasets. Qualitative data are only available in their original language.

France

The Qualitative Social Science Survey Bank (beQuali) is part of the DIME-SHS (Data, Infrastructures, Methods in HSS) excellence facility. It was developed at the Centre for Sociopolitical Data and was started in 2011.

Germany

In 2011 Germany instituted a data service for qualitative data, Quali Service. The archive houses interview data from the Life-Course Achieve (ALLF) at the University of Bremen (Medjedović & Witzel, 2010/2011).

Hungary

In 2009 the Hungarian State Research Fund help support Voices of the 20th Century-Archive and Research Center (Voices). Voices developed a public archive of existing qualitative data collected in Communist and post-Communist periods.

Ireland

The Irish Qualitative Data Archive (IQDA) is a complementary service to the leading center in Ireland for archiving qualitative data, the Irish Social Science Data Archive (ISSDA). The IQDA was founded in 2008 at the National Institute for Regional and Spatial Analysis at the National University of Ireland, Maynooth. It is the national repository of qualitative data generated in or about Ireland (Geraghty, 2014). Regarding applicants for state funding the Irish Research Council (2013) asked the researchers to "specify the means by which that data will be made available as a public good for use by other researchers" (p. 15). The IQDA has a publication that is freely available called Best Practice in Archiving Qualitative Data (Gray, Komolafe, O'Byrne, O'Carroll, & Murphy, 2011). It includes step-by-step guidelines for designing, collecting, and preparing qualitative data for posterity. This Best Practice publication came about through the collaboration of the IQDA with Tallaght West Childhood Development Initiative which focused on developing an archiving strategy for qualitative data obtained from CDI service evaluations (Geraghty, 2014). The Best Practice in Archiving Qualitative Data provides valuable advice for researchers, for example, in developing an archiving strategy appropriate to the level of sensitivity.

Gray and O'Carroll (2010/2011) reported that all new qualitative data in the social sciences collected within the Irish Social Science Platform (www.issplatform.ie) will be made available online through the IQDA. Some longitudinal projects with qualitative components include:

• Growing up in Ireland: Qualitative Module of the National Longitudinal Study on Children
• Life histories and social change in 20th century Ireland
• The process of youth homelessness: A qualitative longitudinal cohort study
• Migrant careers and aspirations
• Women's oral history project
• Leaving school in Ireland
• Irish Centre for Migration Studies Life Narratives Collection

Australian Data Archive

The Australian Data Archive (ADA) provides a national service for collecting and preserving digital research data. These data are available for secondary analysis by researchers. The ADA was established in 1981 and is managed by the Australian National University. The ADA consists of sub-archives: Social Science, Historical, Indigenous, Longitudinal, Qualitative, Crime & Justice, and International.

The ADA qualitative sub-archive is managed by a team of qualitative researchers at the University of Queensland and the University of Sydney. Other universities in Australia provide a wider reference panel: University of Melbourne, University of Technology Sydney, the University of Western Australia, and the Australian National University. The ADA Qualitative archives digital qualitative data generated through social science research. It specializes in primary data collected through interviews, observation, focus groups, or other qualitative data collecting methods instead of existing written texts or historical records. This sub-archive does not store non-digital data like audio or video cassettes or hand-written field notes. The ADA Qualitative provides guidelines for researchers in designing a project methodology based on secondary data analysis.

Data repository guidelines

Antes, Walsh, Strait, Hudson-Vitale, and Dubois (2018) examined data repository guidelines for qualitative data sharing. They separately coded two types of qualitative data repository guidelines: one for primary researchers who want to deposit their data and one for researchers wishing to conduct secondary analysis of the archived data. The purpose was to review English language repository guidelines that accept social science datasets or multidisciplinary datasets. Thirty-two English language social science data repositories were located of which 11 had no qualitative data sharing guidelines, leaving 12 with guidelines for qualitative data. These repositories were across the globe from the U.S. to Czech, to Swiss, Norwegian, and Slovenian guidelines. The length of the guidelines varied from a 2-page document to a series of 11 documents that totaled 122 pages.

Antes et al. (2018) identified three main categories of topics in the guidelines: participant protections, documentation to be submitted, and fees (Table 7.3). Eleven of the twelve repositories offered researchers depositing their data the option to embargo sharing their dataset for a specified period of time and addressed the need for metadata describing the files. Ten of the twelve repositories addressed access levels for the dataset which permitted researchers depositing their data to specify open access or some restrictions to accessing the data. Only half of the guidelines focused on navigating ethical issues such as providing an anonymization log.

Issues addressed in the guidelines for secondary use of the archived dataset included two categories: published requirements before access (why requesting the data) and after access (restrictions of use of data) (Antes et al., 2018) (Table 7.4). All 12 repositories required secondary data analysts to cite the data source in publications. Ten of the twelve guidelines allowed restricted access terms. All 12 repositories required secondary users to promise to maintain data anonymity. Nine of the twelve repositories required additional requirements of researchers wanting access to dataset, such as explaining how data would be used and prohibiting redistribution of the dataset to other users.

Antes et al. (2018) found that only 38% of social science data repositories included guidelines for depositing data and secondary use of the qualitative data. In their content analysis they identified gaps in topics included in the guidelines. Only half of the repository guidelines asked for an anonymization log which documents the steps researchers used to delete direct identifiers. This information would provide important context for secondary users. Another apparent gap was that though 10 of the 12 guidelines addressed deleting direct identifiers only half of the repositories mentioned deleting or replacing indirect identifiers. Only a little over half of the guidelines addressed requesting proof of permission or a waiver to share the dataset with other researchers.

Antes et al. (2018) made some recommendations based on their findings from their content analysis of qualitative data repositories. They recommend qualitative researchers contact institutional and repository representatives from the very beginning of their research studies. In the earliest stages of planning for IRBs for human subject protection and the informed consent, qualitative researchers

TABLE 7.3 Topics addressed in data-depositing guidelines

Topic	1	2	3	4	5	6	7	8	9	10	11	12	%
Participant protections													
Anonymization: Remove or replace direct identifiers	✓	✓	–	✓	–	✓	✓	✓	✓[a]	✓	✓	✓	83
Anonymization: Remove or replace indirect identifier	–	✓	–	–	–	–[b]	✓[c]	✓[a]	✓	✓	✓	✓	50
Anonymization log	–	–	–	–	–	–	✓	✓	✓	✓	✓	✓	50
Set access controls: Specify if access is restricted (and how)	✓	✓	✓	✓	✓	–	–[b]	✓	✓	✓	✓	✓	83
Set access controls: Dissemination is delayed (embargo)[d]	✓	✓	✓	✓	–	✓	✓	✓	✓	✓	✓	✓	92
Adhere to requirements of ethics committee (e.g. IRB, REC)	✓	✓	✓	✓	–	–	–	–[b]	✓	–	✓	✓	58
Proof or waiver of REC permissions for archiving	✓	✓	✓	✓	–	–	✓	✓	✓	✓	✓	✓	83
Proof or waiver of REC permissions for sharing/regulating access	–	–	✓	✓	–	–	✓	✓	–[b]	–	✓	✓	50
Documents to be submitted													
Research methods and practices	✓	✓	–	✓	–	–	✓	✓	✓	✓	✓	✓	75
Data collection instruments	✓	✓	–	✓	–	–	✓	✓	✓	✓	✓	✓	75
Data collection process/approach and problems	✓	✓	–	✓	–	–	–	✓	✓	✓	✓	✓	67
Codebook	✓	✓	–	✓	–	–	–	✓	✓	✓	✓	✓	67
Data documentation/metadata	✓	✓	–	✓	✓	✓	✓	✓	✓	✓	✓	✓	92
Bibliography	✓	✓	✓	✓	–	–	✓	✓	✓	✓	✓	✓	83
Liability Waver	✓	–	–	✓	✓	✓	✓	–	✓	✓	✓	✓	75
DDI-compliance/clearly labeling data files	✓	✓	–	–	✓	✓	✓	✓	✓	–	✓	✓	75
Fees													
Fee required for depositing some or all data files[e]	–	–	–	–	–	✓	–	✓	✓	–	–	–	25

Note: 1 = Australian Data Archive; 2 = Slovenian Science Data Archives; 3 = Czech Social Science Data Archive MEDARD Catalog; 4 = Databrary at New York University and Penn State; 5 = Dataverse U.S. Murray Research Center at Harvard; 6 = The Dryad Repository at North Carolina State University; 7 = Swiss Centre of Expertise in the Social Sciences; 8 = Finnish Social Sciences Data Archive; 9 = Inter-University Consortium for Political and Social Research at the Institute for Social Research at the University of Michigan; 10 = Norwegian Social Science Data Services; 11 = Qualitative Data Repository at Syracuse; 12 = U.K. Data Archive; Π = guidelines address topic; – = no mention of topic in guidelines; IRB = institutional review board; REC = research ethics committee; DDI = Data Documentation Initiative.

a Repository requires vaguer descriptors but discourages pseudonyms and fictionalizations.

b Repository contract indicated that the topic is addressed internally rather than in the written guidelines.

c Repository discourages removing or replacing indirect identifiers.

d Delaying is an available option for depositing researchers but not required for deposit.

e Some repository contacts mentioned fees for depositors, but these were not written in the guidelines.

Reprinted with permission from Antes et al. (2018, p. 67).

TABLE 7.4 Topics addressed in secondary data use guidelines

Topic	1	2	3	4	5	6	7	8	9	10	11	12	%
Published requirements before access													
Complete application to access data	✓	✓	–	✓	–	–	–[a]	✓	✓	✓	✓	✓	67
Clarification given about potential fees	✓	✓	✓	–	–	✓	✓	✓	✓	–	–	✓	67
Data producer permission for some or all datasets	✓	✓	✓	✓	✓	–	✓	✓	✓	–	✓[b]	✓	83
Fulfill special conditions to access restricted use data[c]	✓	✓	–	✓	✓	–	✓	✓	✓	✓	✓	✓	83
Justify purpose for data use	✓	✓	–	–	✓	–	✓	✓	✓	✓	✓	✓	75
Adherence to the requirements of research ethics committee	–	✓	–	✓	–	–	–	–	✓	–	–	–	25
After access topics													
Time limit on data use	–	–	–	–	–	–	–[a]	✓	–[a]	✓	–	–[a]	17
Commercial use prohibited	✓	✓	✓	✓	–	✓	✓	✓	✓	–	✓	–[a]	75
Continued data anonymity required	✓	✓	✓	✓	✓	–	✓	✓	✓	✓	✓	✓	92
Redistribution of downloaded data prohibited	✓	✓	✓	✓	–	–	✓	✓	✓	✓	✓	✓	83
Cite data source in publications	✓	✓	✓	✓	✓	✓	✓	✓	✓	✓	✓	✓	100
Secondary user accountable for new discoveries	✓	–	✓	–	✓	✓	✓	✓	–	✓	–[a]		58
Send citations or notify repository about publications written on the basis of the downloaded data	–	✓	✓	–	–	–	✓	✓	–[a]	✓	✓	✓	58
Share new datasets created from secondary use	–	✓	–	–	–	–	–	–	–	–	✓	✓	25

Note: 1 = Australian Data Archive; 2 = Slovenian Science Data Archives; 3 = Czech Social Science Data Archive MEDARD Catalog; 4 = Databrary at New York University and Penn State; 5 = Dataverse U.S. Murray Research Center at Harvard; 6 = The Dryad Repository at North Carolina State University; 7 = Swiss Centre of Expertise in the Social Sciences; 8 = Finnish Social Sciences Data Archive; 9 = Inter-University Consortium for Political and Social Research at the Institute for Social Research at the University of Michigan; 10 = Norwegian Social Science Data Services; 11 = Qualitative Data Repository at Syracuse; 12 = U.K. Data Archive; Π = Guidelines address topic; – = No mention of topic in guidelines.
a   Repository contact indicated that the topic is addressed internally rather than in the written guidelines.
b   Depositors grant Inter-University Consortium for Political and Social Research permission to handle/ disseminate the data.
c   Examples include affiliation with an institution that is a member of the repository or lead researcher status.
Reprinted with permission from Antes et al. (2018, p. 69).

need to make appropriate preparations for data archiving and sharing. Receiving permissions from participants for data archiving and sharing is much easier during the initial informed consent. Participants' preferences regarding use of their qualitative data would be important to know. Do participants wish to be associated with their responses?

In summary, this chapter started with discussing the research data life cycle which extends the research process to archiving qualitative data for reuse by other researchers. Qualitative data archives across the globe were identified. This chapter concluded with data repository guidelines and secondary data use guidelines. In Chapter 8, metaphor analysis as a type of secondary qualitative analysis is covered.

References

Antes, A. L., Walsh, H. A., Strait, M., Hudson-Vitale, C. R., & Dubois, J. M. (2018). Examining data repository guidelines for qualitative data sharing. *Journal of Empirical Research on Human Research Ethics, 13*, 61–73.

Cízek, T. (2010/2011). Archiving qualitative and qualitative longitudinal social sciences data in the Czech Republic. *IASSIST Quarterly, 34/35*, 30–35.

Corti, L., Van den Eynden, V., Bishop, L., & Woollard, M. (2014). *Managing and sharing research data: A guide to good practice*. London: Sage Publications.

DDI Alliance. (2017). Data documentation initiative. Retrieved from http://www.ddialliance.org

Elman, C., & Kapiszewski, D. (2013). *A guide to sharing qualitative data*. Qualitative Data Repository (QDR), Center for Qualitative and Multi Method Inquiry (CQMI), Syracuse University, v1.3 2013-11-05.

Geraghty, R. (2014). Attitudes to qualitative archiving in Ireland: Findings from a consultation with the Irish Social Science Community. *Studia Socjologiczne, 3* (214).

Gray, J., & O'Carroll, A. (2010/2011). Qualitative research in Ireland: Archiving strategies and development. *IASSIST Quarterly, 34/35*, 18–22.

Gray, J., Komolafe, J., O'Byrne, H., O'Carroll, A., & Murphy, T. (2011). Best practice in archiving qualitative data. *NIRSA Working Paper Series No.65*, January 2011.Irish Research Council. (2013). Government of Ireland Research Project Grants Scheme 2013 terms and conditions. Retrieved from http://research.ie/sites/default/files/irc_rpg_2013_terms_conditions_final_converted_online_fixed_link.pdf

Lana, J., Heus, P., & Mulcahy, T. (2008). Data access in a cyber world: Making use of cyber infrastructure. *Transactions of Data Privacy, 1*(1), 2–16.

Medjedović, I., & Witzel, A. (2010/2011). Sharing and archiving qualitative and qualitative longitudinal research data in Germany. *IASSIST Quarterly, 34/35*, 42–46.

Moravcsik, A. (2010). Active citation: A precondition for replicable qualitative research. *PS: Political Science and Politics, 43*(1), 29–35.

Neale, B. (2013). The Timescapes Archive: A resource for qualitative longitudinal research. Retrieved from www.timescapes.leeds.ac.uk?assets/files/arcive/The_timescapes_archive_report

Neale, B., & Bishop, L. (2012). The Timescapes archive: A stakeholder approach to archiving qualitative longitudinal data. *Qualitative Research, 12*, 53–65.

Neale, B., Henwood, K., & Holland, J. (2012). Researching levels through time: Introduction to the Timescapes approach. *Qualitative Research, 12*, 4–15.

Phillippi, J., & Lauderdale, J. (2018). A guide to field notes for qualitative research: Context and conversation. *Qualitative Health Research, 28*, 381–388.

Secure Data Service (SDS). (2011). Access to the Secure Lab UK Data Service. Retrieved from http://www.UKdataservice.ac.UK/get-data/how-to-access/accesssecurelab

Smioski, A. (2010/2011). Establishing a qualitative data archive in Austria. *IASSIST Quarterly, 34/35*, 30–35.

8

METAPHOR ANALYSIS AS A CREATIVE APPROACH FOR SECONDARY QUALITATIVE DATA ANALYSIS

In this chapter, metaphorical analysis as one approach to secondary qualitative data analysis is discussed. Two main approaches for metaphor analysis are described: Metaphor Identification Procedure and the Three-step Metaphor Analysis. Examples from metaphor analyses I have conducted using my primary datasets of traumatic childbirth are presented as illustrations of this technique that is available to qualitative secondary analysts. Ending the chapter is a metaphor example from qualitative researchers in Norway.

Metaphorical analysis

A valuable, but not common, type of qualitative secondary data analysis is metaphor analysis. In the past, metaphors were viewed as of peripheral interest. Now, however, metaphors are seen as central to provide understanding. A metaphor is defined as "a way of conceiving one thing in terms of another, and its primary function is understanding abstract, emotional or other experiences" (Lakoff & Johnson, 1980, p. 36). It is when a metaphor is linked to its experiential basis that it is able to deepen our understanding. Lakoff and Johnson developed the cognitive linguistic approach to metaphors. According to this approach by means of metaphors we are able to understand one conceptual domain in terms of another conceptual domain. These two domains are known as source and target domains. The source domain is where the metaphorical expressions come from, which aid us in understanding the target domain. Lakoff and Johnson use the formula A IS B to characterize a metaphor. A is the target domain and B is the source domain. A is helped to be understood by B. The more the source domain differs from the target domain the more effective the metaphor is. The capitalized 'IS' is shorthand for a collection of experiences on which the metaphor is based. An example of this formula is provided from this author's metaphor analysis of post-traumatic stress disorder (PTSD) after childbirth: PTSD due to childbirth IS a dangerous ocean (Beck, 2016).

Metaphors assist the mind in freedom of expression, which helps us speak to deep experiences. The strength of a metaphor is that is gives something a different life as it helps to capture the essence of an experience. Atkinson (2013) described metaphors as doorways that have major transformational potential. Metaphors "allow us to pass through and traverse beyond self-deception into areas of truthful mindscapes-perhaps to a place where we often dare not to go" (p. 9).

Lakoff and Johnson (1980) identified different types of metaphors. There is not just one type of metaphor. Structural metaphors allow a highly structural and clearly portrayed concept to structure another concept. Orientational metaphors helps organize an entire system of concepts with respect to one another. Most often orientational metaphors involve spatial orientation such as up and down and in and out. Ontological metaphors have their basis in our experiences with physical objects including our own bodies. Two examples of ontological metaphors are personification and container metaphors. Personification metaphors help to understand a phenomenon in the world in human terms. Here something that is not human is perceived by means of a metaphor as assuming human qualities. An example of a personification metaphor comes again from the author's metaphor analysis of PTSD after birth trauma. One of Beck's (2016) metaphors was PTSD after birth IS a thief in the night. With container metaphors one imposes a boundary, even when there is no boundary present, to mark off or divide an inside and an outside. One example of this metaphor type is PTSD after birth IS an invisible wall.

Inexpressibility, vividness, and compactness are three properties of metaphors (Ortony, 1993). Metaphors give form to some aspect of an experience that is inexpressible. Vividness is accomplished by metaphors using everyday concrete language which helps making intangible experiences more tangible. In their compactness, metaphors include a large degree of information into a compact package.

In the health and social sciences metaphor analysis can provide valuable insights. Metaphorical expressions open up a space for persons to explain what they are experiencing. When a metaphor is understood, something new is created (Ortony, 1993). Metaphors can be used, for instance, by patients to articulate their everyday experiences of their illness. Patients can communicate more effectively with their health-care providers in ways that cannot be captured by unfamiliar medical terminology. Two approaches that secondary analysts can use to conduct a metaphor analysis are described here. First is the Metaphor Identification Procedure (Pragglejaz Group, 2007), and second is Steger's (2007) Three-step Metaphor Analysis.

Metaphor identification procedure

Pragglejaz Group is an international group of metaphor researchers who developed an explicit method for identifying metaphors in discourse. The name of the group was created from the initial letters of their first names. The Pragglejaz Group's (2007) Metaphor Identification Procedure includes the following steps:

1   Read the entire text-discourse to establish a general understanding of the meaning.
2   Determine the lexical units in the text discourse.
3   a   For each lexical unit in the text, establish its meaning in context, that is, how it applies to an entity, relation, or attribute in the situation evoked by the text (contextual meaning). Take into account what comes before and after the lexical unit.
    b   For each lexical unit, determine if it has a more basic contemporary meaning in other contexts that the one in the given context. For our purposes, basic meanings tend to be more concrete (what they evoke is easier to imagine, see, hear, feel, smell, and taste); related to bodily action; more precise; and historically older.
    c   If the lexical unit has a more basic current-contemporary meaning in other contexts than the given context, decide whether the contextual meaning contrasts with the basic meaning but can be understood in comparison with it.
4   If yes, mark the lexical unit as metaphorical.

(p. 3)

The three-step metaphor analysis

Steger (2007) developed a three-step process for metaphorical analysis. Step 1 is metaphor identification and selection. In this initial step the researcher needs to gain an overview of the metaphors present in the text. This involves carefully reading and rereading the texts to identify all the metaphors present. Then the researcher needs to choose the outstanding metaphors. Steger offered five different indicators that can help in this identification:

- Repetition involves searching for metaphors that are used multiple times in the text in a similar way.
- Elaboration refers to metaphors that the speaker expanded on by adding details
- Relatedness refers to a metaphor that is used in the context of an important topic in the text. It also means the metaphor summarizes a bigger paragraph.
- Contrast means that the metaphor appears unexpectedly and doesn't seem to fit with the paragraph it is in. Steger also explains contrast as when speakers use an unusual metaphor regarding their social level.
- Emotion fits into the background of an interview and not the text itself. For instance, was the speaker angry when the metaphor was mentioned in the interview?

Step 2 is general metaphor analysis. Here the general meaning of a metaphor is the focus. How do persons understand this metaphor in a wider social group?

The deeper sense of a metaphor in a more general context is examined. Steger provides six tools to help with general metaphor analysis:

- Comparisons—the researcher inquires whether there are alternative metaphors that imply the same thing or are there different contexts where the metaphor could be used.
- Associations—here the researchers can ask if they or other people connect with the metaphor.
- Functions—what is the role of the metaphor being examined? What group of metaphors does this belong to?
- Dimensions—this tool involves reflecting more deeply about the various aspects of the metaphor.
- Categories—this looks at groups of characteristics that a metaphor possesses.
- Concepts—this involves the bigger background of a metaphor. The narrative in which the metaphor appears can be examined.
- Language—here, we need to remember that a metaphor can reflect different cultural patterns. The idiom with which the metaphor is connected is important.

Step 3 is text-immanent metaphor analysis. In this step, the researcher returns to the original text to examine the implications of the metaphor in "its specific context." In this third step Steger (2007) calls on the researcher's creativity to obtain a deeper understanding of the metaphor. As Davidson (1978) reminded us "understanding a metaphor is as much a creative endeavor as making a metaphor" (p. 29). Steger suggested five tools to help with this step:

- Individual comprehension—the focus here is on how the speakers personally perceive the metaphor.
- Individual background—here, we look at the person's closer environment, specifically their position in an organization.
- Individual path—this refers to the speaker's biography and whether the metaphor is typical of a certain person at more than one time.
- Self-concept—here, one examines the deeper structure of the speaker. Does the metaphor tell us something about how the speakers conceptualize themselves?
- Intentions—this focuses on the speaker's conscious or unconscious intentions behind the metaphor.

Examples of Beck's metaphor analyses

I have published three metaphor analyses, which I will briefly describe to provide some examples of this form of qualitative secondary data analysis. All three of these metaphorical analyses can be classified as Thorne's (2013) analytic expansion type of secondary analysis. The Metaphorical Identification Procedure (MIP;

Pragglejaz Group, 2007) was used to analyze the datasets. To comb through a qualitative dataset to find metaphors is really fun and enlightening to you as the researcher. The metaphors you will locate in your participants' narratives are not buried at all, but once you are specifically looking for metaphors, they readily appear. Not every qualitative dataset will have enough metaphors to do this type of secondary analysis. I originally had envisioned doing my first metaphor analysis with the data from my phenomenological study on birth trauma. The findings of mothers' experiences of a traumatic childbirth were powerful and I assumed they would have used some metaphors in describing their births. When I reviewed the dataset, however, there were not enough metaphors to conduct a secondary analysis. I then moved on to a different qualitative dataset on PTSD following birth trauma, which turned out to be rich with metaphors.

An example of one of the steps in the Metaphor Identification Procedure to identify metaphors in women's descriptions of their experiences of PTSD after birth trauma follows to provide a concrete illustration of this step: (Beck, 2016, p. 79)

> Mostly/ from/ the/ time/ he/ was/ born/ right/ up/ until/ recently/ I/ was/ like/ a/ robot/. I/ think/ I/ am/ a/ bad/ mother/ because/ I'm/ a/ mechanical/ mother/ to/ him/.
>
> Out of the 30 lexical units in these two sentences, two lexical units were judged as being used metaphorically: "robot" and "mechanical". Once all the lexical units were identified in the corpus, they were sorted into the metaphors most often used by mothers to describe their PTSD.

Nine metaphors emerged from this qualitative dataset. Counts for each of the nine metaphors were calculated to identify their order of frequency. In Table 8.1 are examples of three of the nine metaphors. Listed under each metaphor are selected examples of phrases women used in their narratives that were grouped together to identify that particular metaphor.

The value of this type of qualitative secondary analysis became very apparent to me as both a researcher and a clinician. These nine metaphors used by mothers provided rich insight into their day-to-day lives that could not be captured by medical jargon. Metaphors gave a new voice to mothers' experiences of PTSD after their traumatic births. Clinicians can listen intently to see if new mothers use any of these metaphors in describing how they feel after giving birth. These metaphors can help to screen women for post-traumatic stress symptoms.

Beck's (2017a) metaphor analysis of mothers' caring for a child with an obstetric brachial plexus injury (OBPI) is another example of this type of qualitative secondary data analysis. My primary dataset came from a phenomenological study where 23 mothers described their experiences providing care to their children with this birth injury (Beck, 2009). The new research question for this secondary qualitative data analysis was "What are the metaphorical expressions used by mothers to describe their experiences caring for their children with obstetric

TABLE 8.1 Selected examples of phrases in three metaphors used by mothers describing PTSD

---

1 PTSD due to childbirth IS a mechanical robot
   a I just went into emotional blankness, sort of stunned silence caring for my baby.
   b I look and act like a zombie: I sometimes go into the bathroom and cry when I cannot hold it in anymore.
   c I would look at my hands and wonder if they were a part of me after all.
   d I think I am a bad mother because I 'm a mechanical mother to my son.
   e I am numb and detached from everything even my baby. I was like a robot going through the motions required looking after my daughter.
   f I looked like my soul had left me and I was an empty shell.
2 PTSD due to childbirth IS a ticking time bomb
   a I have to grit my teeth, almost crying to get through fighting memories of the birth that want to explode inside me.
   b My first year of my baby's life was one of trying to stay clear of emotional landmines.
   c I have blown some mental fuses as a result of the power surges.
   d Trying not to boil over every day. Trying to keep a lid on it.
   e I would absolutely spew my anger at times during the day.
   f To live daily with the fact that you were like a time bomb ready to go off was dreadful.
3 PTSD due to childbirth IS a video on constant replay
   a Every detail of what happened during the birth runs in my mind like a movie.
   b I would replay the birth over and over in my mind and could never get the feelings to resolve or get it to end.
   c Often I woke up sweating and trembling and feeling panicky. Then the video loop would start again.
   d The last 20 minutes or so before my baby was born played over and over again in my head for a year.
   e No one sees the loop tract that runs when I close my eyes and watch my "movies'.
   f It was like having a picture in the TV screen going on all the time without my having any say or control.

---

brachial plexus injuries?" This research question had not been envisioned by myself when I conducted the original phenomenological study. The type of secondary qualitative analysis I used was Thorne's (2013) analytic expansion. In a metaphor analysis the collection of texts that come from natural language use is called a corpus (Charteris-Black, 2004). The corpus for this secondary analysis consisted of 132 pages of typed transcripts for mothers' experiences caring for their children with an OBPI. Out of this sample of 23 mothers, 21 women used metaphors to help articulate their experiences. Seven metaphors were identified in this secondary analysis: a heavy weight, a maze, a juggling act, a simmering pot, a dagger to the heart, a rollercoaster, and a constant battle. Heavy weight was the metaphor with the largest frequency count while fighting battles had the smallest frequency count. The majority of these seven metaphors were structural metaphors. The metaphor of a simmering pot was a container metaphor and the rollercoaster an orientational metaphor.

My third secondary analysis of one of my qualitative datasets focused on mothers' yearly anniversary of their traumatic childbirth (Beck, 2017b). The sample from the primary phenomenological study included 37 mothers. Women from the United States, New Zealand, Australia, and the United Kingdom participated in this electronic survey. Individual narratives provided by the sample ranged from 1 to 19 pages in length for a corpus of 162 single-spaced typed pages. Charteris-Black (2012) explained that no one single metaphor can adequately express an experience. He says that metaphors are like a series of brushstrokes. Eight metaphors were identified in this secondary analysis: a great pretender, a lottery, a trigger, a clock watcher, a giant rubber band, a guilt trip, a sea of sadness, and bottled up anger.

Metaphor analysis example from Norway

In Norway, Johannessen, Möller, Haugen, and Biong (2014) conducted a secondary analysis from an original grounded theory study of 20 Norwegian men and women living with young-onset dementia (Johannessen & Möller, 2013). The purposes of this qualitative secondary analysis were (1) to examine and interpret metaphors used by persons with young-onset dementia in describing their everyday experience, and (2) to compare these results with the original results to determine if this secondary analysis added new knowledge to this topic. Secondary analysis revealed three metaphors: sliding away, leaving traces, and all alone in the world. Sliding away captured the bodily and social aspects of the participants' dementia. Leaving traces concerned how the person with young-onset dementia experienced stigma. The third metaphor, all alone in the world, focused how the participants created some meaning in their daily life. In combining these three metaphors Johannessen et al. identified a shifting sense of being as the core metaphor. Comparing the secondary analysis results with those of the original study did add a deeper knowledge in a more existential way.

In summary, metaphor analysis as one type of secondary qualitative data analysis was described. The Metaphor Identification Procedure and the Three-Step Metaphor Analysis were the two methods chosen to present in this chapter for conducting a metaphor analysis. Examples of metaphor analyses I have done with my original datasets of traumatic childbirth were included here to illustrate the process. In Chapter 9, using the secondary qualitative analysis to develop theory will be addressed.

References

Atkinson, M. (2013). *Creating transformational metaphors.* Vancouver, BC: Exalon Publishing Company.

Beck, C. T. (2009). The Arm: There's no escaping the reality for mothers caring for their children with obstetric brachial plexus injuries. *Nursing Research, 58,* 237–245.

Beck, C. T. (2016). Posttraumatic stress disorder after birth: A metaphorical analysis. *MCN: American Journal of Maternal Child Nursing, 41*, 76–83.

Beck, C. T. (2017a). Caring for a child with an obstetric brachial plexus injury: A metaphor analysis. *Journal of Pediatric Nursing, 36*, 57–63.

Beck, C. T. (2017b). The anniversary of birth trauma: A metaphor analysis. *The Journal of Perinatal Education, 26*, 219–228.

Charteris-Black, J. (2004). *Corpus approaches to critical metaphor analysis.* New York: Palgrave Macmillan.

Charteris-Black, J. (2012). Shattering the bell jar: Metaphor, gender, and depression. *Metaphor and Symbol, 27*, 199–216.

Davidson, D. (1978). What metaphors mean. In S. Sacks (Ed.), *On metaphor* (pp. 29–45). Chicago, IL: University of Chicago Press.

Johannessen, A., & Möller, A. (2013). Experiences of persons with early onset dementia in everyday life: A qualitative study. *Dementia, 12*, 410–424.

Johannessen, A., Möller, A., Haugen, P. K., & Biong, S. (2014). A shifting sense of being: A secondary analysis and comparison of two qualitative studies on young-onset dementia. *International Journal of Qualitative Studies on Health and Well-being, 9*, 24756. doi:10.3402/ghw.v9.24756

Lakoff, G., & Johnson, M. (1980). *Metaphors we live by.* Chicago, IL: University of Chicago Press.

Ortony, A. (1993). *Metaphors and thoughts.* New York: Cambridge University Press.

Pragglejaz Group. (2007). MIP: A method for identifying metaphorically used words in discourse. *Metaphor and Symbol, 22*, 1–39.

Steger, T. (2007). The stories metaphors tell: Metaphors as a tool to describe tacit aspects in narrative. *Field Methods, 19*, 3–23.

Thorne, S. (2013). Secondary qualitative data analysis. In C. T. Beck (Ed.), *Routledge international handbook of qualitative nursing research* (pp. 393–416). New York: Routledge.

9

THEORY DEVELOPMENT USING SECONDARY QUALITATIVE DATA ANALYSIS

The use of secondary qualitative analysis for theory development is the focus of this chapter. Secondary analysts to date have not frequently reused primary datasets for this purpose. It is a fruitful approach that needs to garner more attention. The chapter begins with early examples of secondary analysis of qualitative datasets for theory development. Examples of concept and theory development using qualitative secondary analysis are included in this chapter. Theoretical coalescence is one method for developing middle range theory from a series of qualitative primary studies (Morse, 2018) and is described here. The chapter ends with an example of the development of my own midrange theory of traumatic childbirth using my own multiple primary qualitative datasets.

Although theory building is often described as the ultimate goal of qualitative research, Morgan (2018) in his review of articles in *Qualitative Health Research* revealed that themes are the typical format for reporting qualitative results. Secondary analyses of primary qualitative studies on a similar topic can help to achieve this goal of theory development. Morse (2018) argues that qualitative researchers have only partially fulfilled the goal of qualitative research to develop concepts and theories. To date most qualitative theories are descriptive and context bound instead of being abstract and explanatory. Theoretical coalescence, on the other hand, can be a strategy for analysis of complex concepts and the development of generalizable qualitative theory. Reanalyzing qualitative data from multiple sources in a program of research and comparing and contrasting data in varying contexts and situations can lead to a higher level and a more abstract description of a concept or development of a qualitative theory.

Early examples of theory development using secondary qualitative analysis

Back in 1988 Thorne and Robinson highlighted the use of secondary analysis of multiple qualitative datasets for theory development. These researchers combined two datasets. The first dataset was derived from a qualitative study on the meaning of hospitalization for patients of chronically ill children (Robinson, 1985). The second reanalyzed dataset came from Thorne's (1985) qualitative study on the experiences of families having an adult member with cancer. Both of these studies revealed a common theme of the meaning of health-care relationships in chronic illness. Their secondary analysis yielded a conceptualization of health-care relationships that provided direction for theory development. This conceptualization revealed a three-stage process of naive trusting, disenchantment, and guarded alliance. Their secondary qualitative analysis provided insight into the dynamics of ongoing interactions with persons with chronic illness and their health-care providers.

Concepts are often called the building blocks of theory. Secondary analysis of qualitative datasets can be one approach for concept analysis. Describing the components and characteristics of the concept of hope was the purpose of Volume and Farris's (2000) secondary qualitative analysis. The primary dataset consisted of transcripts from interviews with women who used prescribed anorexiant medications to lose weight. Reuse of the data revealed that hope grew throughout women's weight loss but peaked once the medications were discontinued. Volume and Harris reported that characteristics of hope in these women were different from those of hope found in other contexts.

Qualitative datasets from two primary studies were combined for reuse of these data to form a conceptual foundation of the complex phenomenon of everyday self-care decision making in chronic illness (Thorne, Paterson, & Russell, 2003). The first primary dataset came from a study on Type 1 diabetes while the second primary dataset focused on persons with Type 2 diabetes, HIV/AIDS, and multiple sclerosis. This secondary analysis revealed that conceptualizing self-care decision making in chronic illness is far more complex than simply learning and complying with therapeutic interventions.

Lutz and Bowers (2005) concluded at that time that current models in the literature were not adequate regarding how persons with disabilities perceived their disability and how it influenced their lives. These secondary analysts combined three datasets to help remedy this gap in the literature. Their findings expanded the concept of disability by situating it within the context of the daily lives of individuals with disabilities. Important conceptual conditions of environment, time, and experience were noted. The degree to which persons with disabilities were able to integrate their disability into their everyday lives depended on three factors: effect of their disabling condition, other peoples' perception of disability, and the need and use of resources. Based on their secondary analysis, Lutz and Bowers called for a person-centered model that captures persons' integration of their disability into daily life.

Theoretical coalescence

Synthesizing multiple studies in a program of research through secondary analysis provides what Morse (2001) called incremental evidence. It is by means of this systematic layering of findings that researchers become more certain of their results and this provides an expanding or new perspective that can be used for theory development. Using completed qualitative studies as data increases the context of the original works yielding a stronger and wider theory. Morse (2017) developed theoretical coalescence as a method of combining a series of qualitative studies to create a higher-level theory with increasing scope and complexity. Morse viewed synthesis of multiple qualitative studies, which provides different perspectives, as a "3D" vision on the topic. Different age groups, cultures, times, etc. can be included in this series of qualitative studies.

In conducting theoretical coalescence to develop qualitative theory, it is essential that raw data from various original studies are available for reanalysis. Metasyntheses do not incorporate raw datasets from original studies and therefore Morse calls this type of work "primarily confirmatory label smoothing with limited innovative model or theory building" (Morse, 2018, p. 178). Theoretical coalescence uses raw data as the main source for analysis instead of categories and themes from published qualitative studies as is done in metasyntheses. Morse (2017) shared that the theoretical coalescence is easier if the researcher developing this theory knows the data intimately, meaning that researcher had conducted the primary qualitative studies. Cognitive sliding then is less likely to be a problem. That is, researchers are less likely to be guessing about meanings and bending interpretations since they were the primary researchers. The process of theoretical coalescence includes

1. Identifying significant concepts.
2. Evaluating the development of the concepts common to each study. This will have probably been conducted as each study was conducted, but, for instance in quantitative studies, this may be so. Do these core concepts need to be present in each study? No—other studies may contribute to other types of knowledge. At this point do not exclude any study that you think may be useful.
3. Diagramming the concepts, and their position overall. Locate each concept for each theory, its level of abstraction, and position on the trajectory (noting the target population and so on). Map the concept in position according to the primary contribution it makes to the overall theory.
4. Identifying the attributes common to each example of the concepts. Open each of the concepts and seek common attributes between the concepts. This will provide some indication about how the concepts interlock and share attributes of characteristics across conceptual boundaries. Link them laterally or horizontally by connecting them according to shared attributes.
5. Developing analytic questions about the nature of the overarching concept, identifying the answers in each study, and the attributes/characteristics of each study.
6. Diagramming and writing the midrange theory (Morse, 2017, pp. 649–650).

The studies included in theoretical coalescence are theoretically connected by sharing characteristics that aid the theory development. There is no deliberate replication. Studies included do not need to overlap. Using a series of qualitative studies overcomes the criticism of small qualitative studies. Morse suggested using in a figure different shapes of the studies included in theoretical coalescence to illustrate the scope, different age groups and populations, and contexts of the studies to present the studies used to create a midrange theory of broader scope than any one qualitative study (Figure 9.1) (Morse, 2017, p. 650).

Morse (2018) provided an example from the qualitative data of her research program on suffering to reanalyze these datasets to focus on the concept of enduring in suffering which had not been the focus of her primary studies. This required secondary analysis of the primary studies included recoding and reinterpreting these datasets. Morse reanalyzed data from 16 of her studies in her development of the concept of enduring.

Using Morse's method of theoretical coalescence, Robinson (2016) developed a middle range theory of trust in health-care relationships in the context of chronic illness. Robinson and Thorne had conducted a series of qualitative studies in the 1980s and 1990s with families experiencing a variety of chronic illnesses. They used secondary analysis of two phenomenological studies and two grounded theory studies. Reanalyzing their qualitative data yielded a grounded theory with three stages of the evolution of trust in interpersonal health-care relationships in chronic illness. Stage 1 was titled Safekeeping, Stage 2 was titled Disenchantment, and Stage 3 was titled Guarded Alliance. During Safekeeping naive trust occurred but was replaced by distrust in the stage of Disenchantment. In the third stage of Guarded Alliance, family members established relationships with chosen clinicians but these relationships were guarded and conditional. Secondary analysis revealed four relationship types in Guarded Alliance that centered on two dimensions of trust:

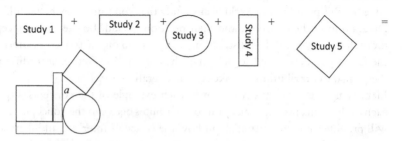

FIGURE 9.1 Placing studies laterally using theoretical coalescence to create a midrange theory of broader scope than any single study.

a, gap, new data needed.

Reprinted with permission from Morse (2017, p. 650).

trust in clinicians and trust in a person's own ability to manage their chronic illness. These four types included hero worship, team playing, resignation, and consumerism.

Middle range theory of Traumatic Childbirth: The Ever-Widening Ripple Effect

Using theoretical coalescence, I conducted a secondary analysis of data from my decade long research program on traumatic childbirth (Beck, 2015). My program of research was predominantly qualitative and included eight phenomenological studies, plus one narrative inquiry, one case study, two mixed methods studies, one qualitative survey, and one prior secondary qualitative analysis. Because I conducted these studies myself, I was privy to the intimate details of the qualitative data and had total access to these datasets which decreased the risk of cognitive sliding.

Diagrammed in Figure 9.2 are the studies along with the different types of groups included in my research program from the population level at top to the obstetric health-care providers at the bottom. Gaps where new data are needed also are included in this diagram.

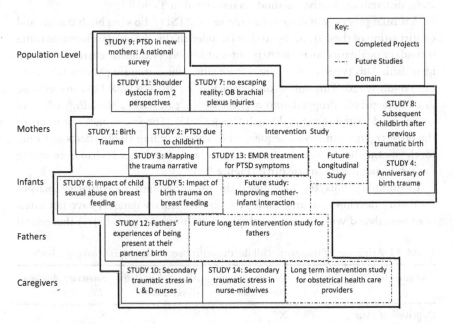

FIGURE 9.2 Research program conducted in the domain of Traumatic Birth Syndrome.

Note: PTSD = post-traumatic stress disorder; OB = obstetric; EMDR = eye movement desensitization reprocessing; L&D = labor and delivery.

Reprinted with permission from Beck (2015, p. 3).

I identified nine axioms for my midrange theory of traumatic childbirth. Two examples are "Traumatic childbirth can have long-term, chronic consequences" and "At the anniversary of a traumatic birth, posttraumatic stress symptoms can flair up" (Beck, 2015, pp. 3–4).

Next analytic questions were asked of the studies themselves:

1. What is it about childbirth that can be so traumatic?
2. What are the essential characteristics of posttraumatic stress due to birth trauma?
3. Are there long-term consequences of birth trauma for the mother?
4. Does a traumatic childbirth affect more than just the mother?
5. What strategies do women use to get through a subsequent pregnancy following a traumatic birth?
6. What is secondary posttraumatic stress due to attending a traumatic birth? (Beck, 2015, p. 4).

The attributes of a traumatic birth included: deprived of caring, stripped of their dignity, terrifying loss of control, neglected communication, and buried and forgotten (Beck, 2015, p. 4). These attributes were confirmed by secondary analysis using different qualitative methods as illustrated in Table 9.1.

A similar process was done for attributes of PTSD following birth trauma and confirmation of these from my studies included in this theory development using secondary qualitative analysis. Attributes of secondary traumatic stress were also identified. This type of stress comes from clinicians caring for patients who have been traumatized. Through secondary qualitative analysis what I discovered was, just like a pebble dropped into a pond which can have a spreading effect of ripples, so does traumatic childbirth (Beck, 2015). The few minutes or hours of the birth trauma can have a sequence of ever expanding ripple effects not only for the mother herself but also for her family, and clinicians who had been caring for her during the traumatic birth (Figure 9.3).

In summary, Chapter 9 discussed the use of secondary qualitative analysis for theory development and concept analysis. Primary datasets have not often been reanalyzed with theory development in mind. Morse's (2018) theoretical

TABLE 9.1 Attributes of traumatic childbirth confirmed by three qualitative methods

Characteristics	Phenomenology (Beck, 2004a)	Narrative Analysis (Beck, 2006a)	Secondary Analysis (Beck, 2013)
Deprived of caring	X	X	X
Stripped of dignity	X	X	X
Terrifying loss of control	X	X	X
Neglected communication	X	X	X
Buried and forgotten	X		

Reprinted with permission from Beck (2015, p. 5).

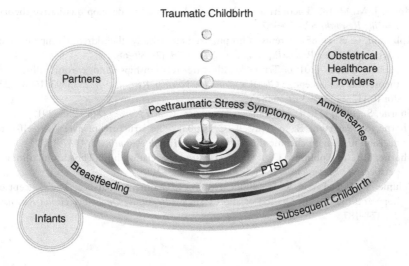

FIGURE 9.3   Middle range theory of Traumatic Childbirth: The Ever-Widening Ripple Effect.

Printed with permission from Beck (2015).

coalescence was concentrated on as a method to develop theory from secondary qualitative analysis. Examples are provided of some secondary analyses that have been conducted to develop qualitative theory, including a middle range theory of mine entitled Traumatic Childbirth: The Ever-Widening Ripple Effect. In Chapter 10, I focus on presenting strategies I have used with my PhD student in my qualitative methods courses to teach secondary qualitative data analysis.

References

Beck, C. T. (2004a). Birth trauma: In the eye of the beholder. *Nursing Research, 53*, 28–35.

Beck, C. T. (2006a). Pentadic cartography: Mapping birth trauma narratives. *Qualitative Health Research, 16*, 453–466.

Beck, C. T. (2013). The obstetric nightmare of shoulder dystocia: A tale of two perspectives. MCN: *The American Journal of Maternal Child Nursing, 38*, 34–40.

Beck, C. T. (2015). Middle range theory of traumatic childbirth: The ever-widening ripple effect. *Global Qualitative Nursing Research.* doi:10.1177/233339361557513

Lutz, B. J., & Bowers, B. J. (2005). Disability in everyday life. *Qualitative Health Research, 15*, 1037–1054.

Morgan, D. L. (2018). Themes, theories, and models. *Qualitative Health Research, 28*, 339–345.

Morse, J. M. (2001). Qualitative verification: Building evidence by extending basic findings. In J. M. Morse (Ed.), *The nature of qualitative evidence* (pp. 203–220). Thousand Oaks, CA: Sage Publication.

Morse, J. M. (2017). Theoretical coalescence. In J. M. Morse (Ed.), *Analyzing and conceptualizing the theoretical foundations of nursing* (pp. 647–651). New York: Springer Publishing Company.

Morse, J. M. (2018). Theoretical coalescence: A method to develop qualitative theory. *Nursing Research, 67,* 177–187.

Robinson, C. A. (1985). Parents of hospitalized chronically ill children: Competency in question. *Nursing Papers/Perspectives in Nursing, 17*(2), 59–68.

Robinson, C. A. (2016). Trust, health care relationships, and chronic illness: A theoretical coalescence. *Global Qualitative Nursing Research, 3,* 2333393616664823. doi:10.1177/2333393616664823

Thorne, S. (1985). The family cancer experience. *Cancer Nursing, 8*(5), 285–291.

Thorne, S., Paterson, B., & Russell, C. (2003). The structure of everyday self-care decision making in chronic illness. *Qualitative Health Research, 13,* 1337–1352.

Thorne, S.E., & Robinson, C.A. (1988). Health care relationships: The chronic illness a perspective. *Research in Nursing & Health, 11,* 293–300.

Volume, C. I., & Farris, K. B. (2000). Hoping to maintain a balance: The concept of hope and the discontinuation of anorexiant medications. *Qualitative Health Research, 10,* 174–187.

10

TEACHING SECONDARY QUALITATIVE DATA ANALYSIS

Preparing the next generation of qualitative researchers brings responsibility to ensure that PhD students are exposed to secondary qualitative analysis and to opportunities to practice reusing datasets under faculty guidance. In teaching, faculty can use their own qualitative datasets or archived ones. This chapter begins with the benefits for students of reanalyzing qualitative datasets. Next the ethics involved in using archived data from a teaching perspective are identified. The majority of this chapter provides three examples of teaching strategies that I have used with my PhD students in the School of Nursing at the University of Connecticut. One example was designed for PhD students' research internships and two of the examples were part of my advanced qualitative research methods course. These are presented here to provide examples of teaching strategies that faculty can use or pattern their own assignments after. The chapter ends with an example of an archive, the U. K. Data Service, which provides teaching opportunities for faculty using its data.

Often, in the beginning, students describe feeling like they are drowning in all the qualitative data. Benefits for students in reusing a qualitative dataset under faculty supervision are many. Students can practice analyzing qualitative data. They can identity new research questions that can be answered by the dataset. Accessibility to a dataset also provides opportunities for students to critique the research design used in the primary study. Students can identify if there are gaps in the dataset that, if this were not a class exercise, they would need to collect additional data to answer their research question.

Bishop (2012) examined the ethical implications of using archived qualitative data for teaching proposes. She brought to the forefront three issues regarding reuse of data for teaching. The first involves weighing the benefits to students' learning needs against the risk of data sharing. The second focuses on giving the opportunity to different qualified groups, such as researchers and students, equitable access to the dataset. The third involves respecting the autonomy of not only the research participants but also the students.

Examples of teaching assignments for qualitative secondary data analysis

The research internship and one of the class assignments in my course used data from a mixed methods study of mine on secondary traumatic stress in labor and delivery nurses (Beck & Gable, 2012). Secondary traumatic stress results from a clinician helping or wanting to help a traumatized or suffering patient (Figley, 1995). Secondary traumatic stress is a syndrome of symptoms clinicians can experience that are similar to post-traumatic stress disorder (PTSD). In the following section I have provided the metadata for this study focusing on the qualitative strand of this mixed methods study. Metadata, data about data, is important for qualitative secondary data analysis because it is an essential form of communication between the primary researchers and the secondary analysts. It provides answers about the original dataset that secondary analysts need to help them have a more complete understanding of the dataset and its context. I have the students read this before they start the assignment to learn about the context of the qualitative dataset they will be privy to. After the students have read the metadata, we meet and discuss any questions they may have about the dataset before they begin their secondary analysis.

Metadata for use with assigments

Secondary Traumatic Stress in Labor and Delivery Nurses: A Mixed Methods Study (Beck & Gable, 2012).

The dataset provided here follows the recommendations of the Inter-university Consortium for Political and Social Science (ICPSR; www.icpsr.umich.edu).

ICPSR lists the following important metadata elements:

- Principal investigator
- Funding sources
- Data collector/producer
- Project description
- Sample and sampling procedures
- Data collection
- Data sources
- Unit of analysis
- Variables
- Data collection instruments

Since this is an example of teaching my PhD students qualitative secondary data analysis, I am concentrating on the qualitative strand of this mixed methods study of secondary traumatic stress in labor and delivery nurses for the metadata. I have described the quantitative instruments used to collect data and also a brief paragraph on quantitative analysis but have not included a list of variables' names and labels. It was not necessary to remove any information in the qualitative data that would allow the research participants to be identified. All data were anonymous. The mixed methods study received exempt status from the University's IRB.

Principal investigator

Cheryl Tatano Beck, DNSc, CNM, FAAN

Funding source

None

Data collector/producer

After obtaining approval from the University's IRB Board and the Association of Women's Health, Obstetric, and Neonatal Nursing (AWHONN), data collection began. A packet of materials regarding the study was sent by postal mail to a random sample of 3,000 labor and delivery nurses who were members of AWHONN. Included in the packet were an information sheet describing the study, the Secondary Traumatic Stress Scale (STSS; Bride, Robinson, Yegidis, & Figley, 2004), a demographic information sheet, and directions for the qualitative strand of the mixed methods study. The nurses returning the completed forms implied their informed consent. All data were anonymous.

Project description

A convergent parallel design was used. It is

> a mixed methods design in which the researcher uses concurrent timing to implement the quantitative and qualitative strands during the same phase of the research process, prioritizes the methods equally, keeps the strands independent during analysis, and mixes the results during the researcher's overall interpretation of the data.
>
> *(Creswell & Plano Clark, 2011, p. 410)*

Research questions

1. What is the prevalence and severity of secondary traumatic stress in labor and delivery nurses due to caring for women during traumatic childbirth?
2. What are the experiences of labor and delivery nurses caring for women during traumatic childbirths?

Sample/sampling procedures

This sample consisted of 464 labor and delivery nurses. The mean age of the sample was 46.70 (SD = 11.04). The age of the youngest nurse was 24 years, and the age of the oldest was 80 years. The mean number of years practicing as a registered nurse was 20.77 (SD = 11.66) with a range from 1 year to 57 years. The sample was homogeneous with 99% female, 91% White, and 80% with a bachelor's degree or higher. The majority of nurses (59%) were staff nurses who identified their job setting as hospital inpatient. Out of the 464 returned surveys, 322 of these nurses (70%) participated in the qualitative strand describing their exposure to patients during traumatic births.

Data collection

Quantitative approach

The Secondary Traumatic Stress Scale (STSS) is a 17-item, Likert-type scale that measures secondary traumatic stress symptoms focusing on clinicians' exposure to caring for traumatized populations (Bride et al., 2004). The scale is composed of three subscales: Intrusion, Avoidance, and Arousal. It was developed so that the items on the scale all focus on the traumatic stressor of exposure to traumatized patients. Clinicians rate how often they experienced each symptom in the past seven days using a 5-point Likert-type response scale ranging from "never" to "very often." Bride (2007) offered the following approach for interpreting total scores on the STSS: less than 28 (little or no secondary traumatic stress), 28–37 (mild), 38–43 (moderate), 44–48 (high), and 49 and above (severe secondary traumatic stress). A cutoff score of 38 indicates at least moderate secondary traumatic stress symptoms.

The STSS can also be used to determine if a clinician screens positive for PTSD using the DSM-IV-TR's criteria (American Psychological Association, 2000). To meet these diagnostic criteria, Bride requires a health-care provider to endorse at least one item on the Intrusion subscale, at least three items on the Avoidance subscale, and at least two items on the Arousal subscale. To be considered endorsed on the STSS, an item needs to be rated 3 or higher ("occasionally," "often," or "very often") for a post-traumatic stress symptom.

Qualitative approach. Obstetric nurses were asked to respond to the following statement: "Please describe in as much detail as you can remember your experiences being present at a traumatic childbirth. Specific examples of points that you are making are extremely valuable. You may describe as many experiences as you wish."

Data analysis

Quantitative approach

Descriptive statistics were used to analyze the quantitative data. The relationships between the secondary traumatic stress levels and the following variables were analyze using *t*-tests and correlations: age, gender, years practicing as an RN, highest education received, ethnic background, primary clinical focus, primary position, and job setting.

Qualitative approach

To analyze the labor and delivery nurses' experiences of exposure to traumatic births Krippendorff's (2004) content analysis method was used. The qualitative dataset consisted of 179 single-spaced typed pages. Krippendorff's analytical technique of clustering was employed to identify data that could be grouped together as a theme by sharing some quality. Dendrograms, which are treelike diagrams, helped visualize the data as they were categorized into theme clusters.

This ends the metadata provided to my students. Next are the exercises based on this metadata.

Teaching assignment: example #1

The first example is the most in-depth assignment. I had two PhD students who needed a research internship, so I designed this assignment for them. It entailed each student reading through the qualitative dataset in the mixed methods study of secondary traumatic stress in labor and delivery nurses to choose a specific type of traumatic childbirth to conduct their secondary qualitative analysis. Located in Table 10.1 is a section of my secondary traumatic stress in labor and delivery nurses' codebook for the one variable labeled "trauma type." This table lists 35 specific types of birth trauma nurses reported being exposed to while caring for their laboring patients. In this exercise, first, the PhD students ran descriptive statistics for the variable, trauma type, to identify which type of trauma would have the most qualitative data for them to conduct their secondary analysis. The five traumas with the highest frequency included:

Trauma	# of Participants
• Infant death	85
• Fetal demise	70
• Maternal death	67
• Shoulder dystocia	60
• Forceps/vacuum extraction	26

The PhD students were privy to the complete dataset of 179 typed single-spaced pages of the labor and delivery nurses' narratives. The type of trauma was linked to the participants' ID number. After reviewing the qualitative dataset, the students decided that one of them would choose infant death and the other student would select fetal demise. Fetal demise is the death of a developing fetus after 20 weeks' gestation. While infant death refers to death of a live born infant during the first 28 days of life. Each student would independently conduct their

TABLE 10.1 Secondary traumatic stress codebook for the variable "trauma type"

Variable Name	Code
Trauma type	1 Infant death
	2 Maternal death
	3 Fetal demise (IUFD)
	4 Shoulder dystocia
	5 C/S started with only local anesthetic
	6 Prolapsed cord
	7 Postpartum hemorrhage
	8 Vacuum extraction
	9 Forceps delivery
	10 Resuscitation of infant
	11 Abruptio placenta
	12 Pulmonary embolism
	13 Head entrapment in breech delivery
	14 Decapacitation
	15 Fetal anomalies
	16 Placenta accreta/vasa previa
	17 Emergency C/S
	18 4° laceration
	19 ↓FHR & MD not in hospital
	20 HELLP/eclampsia/DIC
	21 MD physically abusive
	23 Motor vehicle accident
	24 Amniotic embolism
	25 Cardiac arrest
	26 Hysterectomy
	27 Severely brain damaged infant
	28 Young adolescents
	29 Preterm infants
	30 Precipitous delivery
	31 Thyroid storm
	32 Everted uterus/prolapsed uterus
	33 Aggressive induction
	34 Anencephalic infant
	35 Uterine rupture

secondary analysis and then because the topics both involved nurses' experiences with death, the students would next compare and contrast their findings to see if the timing of the death impacted nurses' experiences. They decided they would publish one article together, describing the results of their combined secondary qualitative analyses.

The type of secondary qualitative analysis the PhD students chose was Thorne's (2013) analytic expansion. Three new research questions guided their analyses:

1. What are the labor and delivery nurses' experiences caring for a mother during fetal death?
2. What are labor and delivery nurses' experiences caring for a mother during an infant death?
3. What are the similarities and differences in nurses' experiences caring for women during a fetal death versus an infant death?

The PhD students used the same qualitative analysis as had been used in the primary study: Krippendorff's (2013) content analysis. The faculty member guided the graduate students during each step of their secondary qualitative analysis and answered any questions the students had concerning the primary study and its context.

In 70 cases the labor and delivery nurses experienced being present in a birth where a fetal death occurred and another 85 cases included the experience being present during an infant death. Out of the total 155 cases, 64 of them only mentioned being present for a perinatal loss but no description of their experience was provided. This left 91 cases which had a rich, detailed description that could be used in the students' secondary analyses. The results of their secondary qualitative data analyses can be found in their published article:

Puia, D.M., Lewis, L., & Beck, C.T. (2013). Experiences of obstetric nurses who are present for a perinatal loss. *Journal of Obstetric, Gynecologic, and Neonatal Nursing, 42*, 321–331.

One of the PhD students, Laura Lewis Foran, reflected on her experience of secondary qualitative analysis during her research internship.

Reflection of a PhD student on her experience with secondary qualitative data analysis

I had the opportunity to conduct a secondary qualitative data analysis with a classmate during a one-semester research internship with Dr. Beck in my graduate program. Dr. Beck had recently collected data and conducted a primary analysis using a mixed-methods design, and we had the chance to use the existing dataset to answer a different qualitative research question. We were able to complete the analysis, write a manuscript, and submit for publication over the course of one semester and the following summer.

Using secondary qualitative analysis allowed me to surpass my personal goals for the research internship. I was able to take ownership of a research study, to work with real data, to produce publishable results, and to have an impact beyond a grade at the end of the rotation. As a graduate student balancing a full time course load and full time employment, I was eager to maximize the efficiency of my learning opportunities. My classmate and I were able to save a significant amount of time by jumping in to a research study at the point of analysis while still feeling responsible for the study as a whole. In other words, it did not feel like we worked on a part of Dr. Beck's research study. Instead, it felt like we used Dr. Beck's data to conduct our own research study from beginning to end. Without using this method, we would have likely only been able to work on a single aspect of someone else's project, or else would have sacrificed quality to make the project fit within our time constraints. Secondary qualitative data analysis let us expedite the research process without compromising rigor.

Several factors facilitated the success of this project. First, Dr. Beck briefed us on the primary study and gave us access to the original IRB application to help us fully understand how the data were collected. In our case, we were conducting a qualitative content analysis of written responses to an open-ended question. Knowledge of the primary study allowed us to be mindful of nuances that might affect responses, such as how participants were recruited and what questions they were asked beyond the one that directly applied to our research question.

Working with the primary researcher also helped me understand the "why's" and the "how's" of the data collection process without having personally collected the data, which was important to me as a student. Through our discussions, I was able to see why Dr. Beck chose to collect written responses versus conducting in-person interviews. I learned why she phrased the open-ended questions the way she did, and I could see first-hand the types of responses that resulted from her data collection design choices. I learned about logistical obstacles when recruiting and strategies to overcome those obstacles. Even though I did not participate in the data collection, all of these questions and learning opportunities arose through my close work with the data during data analysis.

The most challenging part of this project for me was that the content area was not familiar to me prior to this rotation. I was an oncology nurse, and our research question was about perinatal loss in labor and delivery nurses. I was initially intimidated to work outside my comfort zone. Dr. Beck and my classmate, a labor and delivery nurse, helped alleviate my concerns by making themselves available to answer my questions about the content. My classmate took the lead on the review of the literature and identified literature for me to read to gain background information. In many ways, my lack of background knowledge allowed me to stay unbiased. I relied solely on the systematic use of method and the data in front of me to draw conclusions. I learned that if I stayed true to the research method, the content would follow. My classmate and I also brought diverse perspectives to the discussion section, as we approached the data from very different lenses given our clinical backgrounds. After completing this study, I would not hesitate to work on another project outside my content expertise as long as I knew that a content expert was on my research team. Secondary qualitative data analysis offers rich opportunities for students to take charge of their own work and to produce high quality publishable products within condensed time frames. Participating in this project was one of the most enriching experiences in my program of study.

Teaching assignment: example #2

A second type of teaching assignment to provide students with a hands-on experience of secondary analysis with a qualitative dataset involves one that can occur during class time in a qualitative methods course. It is designed to be completed within one class period. If the professor has a qualitative dataset of his/her own, this works best. The professor is privy to all the details of the qualitative study where the dataset is from and can share this as an introduction to the class assignment. Here is one that I have used with my PhD students in an advanced qualitative research methods course at the University of Connecticut.

Researchers often use content analysis in their qualitative secondary analysis. Two different approaches can be used in content analysis for qualitative data. One way is to analyze the data for emerging themes. In the second approach preset categories are used to comb through the data to extract relevant data for a particular category. Since my assignment was to be completed in one class period, I chose content analysis using preset categories. This could be accomplished in a shorter period of time and with fewer narratives than thematic analysis.

Again, I used the dataset from the qualitative strand of my mixed methods study of secondary traumatic stress in labor and delivery nurses (Beck & Gable, 2012). I gave the students the metadata to read prior to the start of the assignment. This time, however, I also gave students the DSM-IV-TR's (2000) diagnostic criteria for post-traumatic stress disorder (PTSD), which included three major categories of symptoms: Intrusions, Avoidance, and Arousal. Intrusions referred to recurrent and intrusive remembering of the distressing events. Avoidance refers to avoiding thoughts, feelings, and places that remind the person of the trauma. Arousal includes symptoms of increased Arousal such as difficulty falling asleep, irritability, anger, and difficulty concentrating. Clinicians experiencing secondary traumatic stress experience similar symptoms as PTSD. I also provided students with a number of the narratives from the qualitative portion of the mixed methods dataset where obstetric nurses described experiencing these symptoms. The students spent the class period conducting qualitative secondary analysis of my dataset using content analysis with the DSM-IV-TR's preset categories of Intrusions, Avoidance, and Arousal. Each student highlighted selected sentences in the narrative and identified whether the labor and delivery nurses were referring to Intrusions, Avoidance, or Arousal. In Table 10.2 are examples of two narratives with the coding for the secondary analysis.

TABLE 10.2 Two narratives of labor and delivery nurses' experiences caring for women during a traumatic birth

Narrative #1 (Infant Death)

I came into work for my 7 am shift. While receiving report, my patient (who I had not met yet) called out at 07:33 am to say her "baby was not breathing" (he was just under 12-hours-old). I ran into her room and her husband handed me a baby who had clearly been dead for quite some time (he was mottled, blue, and cold). We did every resuscitation effort possible, even though we all knew it was futile. After 25 minutes and with the parents' permission, we stopped our efforts. I then cared for these parents the rest of the day. I attended the funeral of their baby, and send them a card on the anniversary of this birth/death (it was on Thanksgiving Day, so very unforgettable).

For the next 5-7 months, I cried constantly, **suffered insomnia**, had **anxiety attacks**, and *had difficulty returning to work* (I returned after a few weeks, but still shake every time I hear the call bell, it's been a year and a half). I also suffered extreme guilt asking myself why I didn't go into the room promptly at 7 am, because maybe, he was still alive then (we always let our patients sleep in until breakfast comes at 08.00 am). I will never, ever be able to forget this trauma. I carry it with me daily. His death was ruled as SIDS, with the possibility of "overlay" (blanket over his face). No other cause was found, and we will never know.

I often feel I have to *emotionally distance myself from patients* because to become emotionally involved, and experience their labor and birth, would completely empty me of emotion and life.

For a while I had a *hard time fully engaging or being present when doing things with my family* because I was always replaying work situations. I would even call into work to make sure that patients I had taken care of were doing ok and that I did not miss anything or forget to do something.

Narrative #2 (Infant Death)

The last traumatic child birth I was involved in was a term delivery of an infant with numerous internal and external anomalies. Before coming to our providers, the patient had gone to a different provider who failed to notify this couple of the anomalies in time for a first semester abortion. This couple had chosen no heroics but to hold their baby girl until the end. At one point during the night, we thought we had lost her, but she suddenly started breathing again. After making it through the night, I went in to her room after my shift to say goodbye to her. It was obvious by the agonized breathing that this infant was having, that she would expire soon. The patient's husband had to attend to the other children, leaving her alone to deal with their baby. I stayed with her until her baby passed. As the heart rate decreased, we sat together on her bed and I just held both of them until it was over, and cried like a baby with the mom. Thank goodness I was off for several days after that because this was very stressful and exhausting.

When I deal with patients experiencing loss as I have, I seem to relive the trauma and will **have trouble sleeping** and go over in my mind all the details of the time period. I find myself *pulling away from other staff*. I don't want to take breaks with them, believing that they will want to talk about our patients and their care for the day.

Narrative #2 (Infant Death)

If a patient has a very hard delivery, I know other staff at the delivery want to talk about what happened but *I just want to be alone and not discuss what happened.* I find myself giving in to my desire to stay in bed the next day if I am off. I also <u>seem to be thinking about the events after and on my way home</u> in the evening. These thoughts are not what went wrong, just what happened and could I have seen or missed something that might have clued me into what would happen.

Bold = Arousal.
<u>Underlining</u> = Intrusions.
Italics = Avoidance.

Teaching assignment: example # 3

The third example of an assignment that can be used to teach students secondary qualitative analysis is designed to alert students to the number of variations of types of secondary analysis that currently are published. Prior to class, I chose a different published qualitative secondary analysis article for each student to review. I tried to find articles that were close to each student's dissertation topic to increase their interest in the assignment. Students were assigned to read the study given to them before the start of the next class and complete the codebook for their study (Appendix C). This was the codebook I used in my review of secondary qualitative analyses conducted in the discipline of nursing that is described in Chapter 12. In the next class, time was provided for students to describe and share the type of secondary qualitative analysis used in their assigned study. Students were surprised at the number of variations across their studies, especially when looking at the primary researcher's relationship to the original dataset.

U.K. Data Service

Some qualitative archives also provide excellent opportunities for teaching. One example is the U.K. Data Service (https://www.ukdataservice.ac.uk). It provides teaching resources for faculty who want to instruct their students in qualitative secondary analysis. Faculty can access datasets specifically designed for teachers and their students. Also, faculty can find ideas for teaching with data exemplars at the U.K. Data Service website. Case studies describing how other faculty have used these resources into their teaching are available. The datasets for teaching by the U.K. Data Service provide students with raw material for secondary analysis. Faculty can also view a video tutorial describing the various resources available for teaching.

In summary, in this chapter, I focused mainly on teaching assignments I have given my doctoral students at the University of Connecticut to provide specific examples. In Chapter 11, general guidelines for writing up and publishing secondary qualitative data analyses are addressed.

References

American Psychological Association. (2000). *Diagnostic and statistical manual of mental disorders – Text revision* (4th ed.). Washington, DC: Author.

Beck, C. T., & Gable, R. K. (2012). Secondary traumatic stress in labor and delivery nurses: A mixed methods study. *Journal of Obstetric, Gynecologic, and Neonatal Nursing, 41*, 747–760.

Bishop, L. (2012). Using archived qualitative data for teaching: Practical and ethical considerations. *International Journal of Social Research Methodology, 15*, 341–350.

Bride, B. E. (2007). Prevalence of secondary traumatic stress among social workers. *Social Work, 52*, 63–70.

Bride, B. E., Robinson, M. M., Yegidis, B., & Figley, C. R. (2004). Development and validation of the Secondary Traumatic Stress Scale. *Research on Social Work Practice, 14*, 27–35.

Creswell, J. W., & Plano Clark, V. L. (2011). *Designing and conducting mixed methods research.* Thousand Oaks, CA: Sage Publications.

Figley, C. R. (1995). Compassion fatigue: Toward a new understanding of the costs of caring. In B. H. Stamm (Ed.), *Secondary traumatic stress: Self-care issues for clinicians, researchers, and educators* (pp. 3–28). Lutherville, MD: Sidran Press.

Krippendorff, K. (2004). *Content analysis: An introduction to its methodology.* Thousand Oaks, CA: Sage Publications.

Krippendorff, K. (2013). *Content analysis: An introduction to its methodology.* Thousand Oaks, CA: Sage Publications.

Puia, D. M., Lewis, L., & Beck, C. T. (2013). Experiences of obstetric nurses who are present for a perinatal loss. *Journal of Obstetric, Gynecologic, and Neonatal Nursing, 42*, 321–331.

Thorne, S. (2013). Secondary qualitative data analysis. In C. T. Beck (Ed.), *Routledge international handbook of qualitative nursing research* (pp. 393–404). New York: Routledge.

11

PUBLISHING SECONDARY QUALITATIVE DATA ANALYSES

In this chapter, general guidelines for publishing secondary qualitative analyses are presented. The structure of this type of secondary analysis journal article is discussed along with suggestions for diagrams and tables that can be used to highlight secondary analysis methods and findings. Figures used in some of my secondary qualitative analyses from my primary datasets are included in this chapter for illustrations.

The focus of this first section is not on the elements of grammar and syntax. There are many excellent books already published that describe these basics of writing. Here the discussion centers specifically on publishing secondary qualitative analyses. Authors always need to remember the audience they have chosen to write for. Is the audience comprised of researchers and academics or clinicians or consumers? Authors should use appropriate secondary analysis terms like analytic expansion or supra analysis but be mindful that readers may not be familiar with these terms so definitions are necessary. Authors can accomplish two aims with their writing. The first is to present the findings of their secondary qualitative analysis, and the second is to educate the reader about this type of research. Some readers may not be familiar with this type of secondary analysis, and a well-written article will educate persons new to this design.

Keywords listed for an article should include secondary qualitative analysis to help identify it for persons searching databases. It also would be a good idea to include this phrase in the title of the article. Full credit and appropriate reference to the primary study should always be included in the article. If the data were obtained from an archive, the name of the archive needs to be specified.

Table 11.1 includes an outline for the structure of a secondary qualitative analysis journal article. Due to the need to describe both the primary and

TABLE 11.1 Structure of a secondary qualitative analysis journal article

Title	State It Is a Qualitative Secondary Analysis
Introduction	• Describe the research problem
	• State significance of the problem for your discipline
Literature review	• Describe and critique relevant research related to topic of secondary analysis
	• Identify the gap in the knowledge your study will fill
Methods	
Primary study	• Purpose
	• Research questions
	• Research design
	• Sample size and type
	• Data collection approaches
	• Data analysis techniques
	• Outcomes
Secondary study	• Source of qualitative dataset: if archival, name specific archive
	• Assessment of quality of dataset
	• Purpose
	• Assessment of fit with purpose of secondary analysis
	• Ethical approval specific for secondary analysis
	• Research questions
	• Research design
	• Secondary data analysis typology used: Thorne, Heaton, Hinds
	• Secondary researcher's relationship to the primary dataset
	• Consultation with primary researcher
	• Samples size and type
	• Data collection
	o Number of datasets used
	o Amount of primary dataset used: entire or subset
	o Any new supplementary data collected
	o Accessibility of data: audio, transcripts, field notes, etc.
	• Data analysis techniques
	• Outcomes

secondary studies, it can be easy for a reader to get confused in the complexity involved in secondary analysis. Blurring of boundaries between the two studies can make it difficult for readers to decide which study is being referred to in that section of the article. For clarity, components of the primary studies need to be clearly identified and kept separate from the components of the secondary studies. Figure 11.1 provides an example of a diagram that can be used. Adding to the challenge of writing a secondary qualitative analysis for a journal is the usual page limitation provided in the author guidelines. Because the description of both the primary and secondary studies needs to be included, this can be problematic. Challenges involved in writing up a

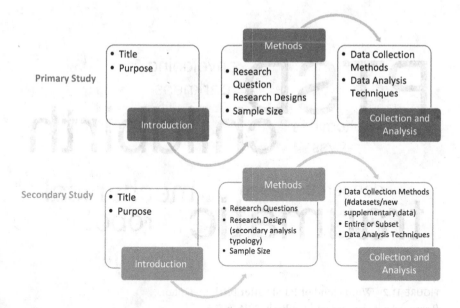

FIGURE 11.1 Diagram for specification of primary and secondary studies' research designs.

secondary qualitative analysis are similar to those for a mixed methods study. In a mixed methods study both strands of the design (qualitative and quantitative) need to be described to fit the constraints of a journal's page count. Authors need to write clearly and concisely so that both the quantitative and qualitative strands are adequately described. Also, each strand needs to be clearly labeled to prevent readers from becoming confused regarding which strand is being referred to in a section of the article; so it is with secondary qualitative analyses. Writing needs to be clear and concise so as to not shortchange the secondary analysis. If the primary study is not described in enough depth, however, the reader cannot assess its fit with the secondary analysis of its data. Inclusion of a diagram of the components and outcomes of both studies can be quite helpful to readers.

In addition to a diagram that presents key elements of both the primary and secondary research designs, tables and figures can be created to highlight the findings of the secondary analysis and provide the grab that is desired in qualitative research. Examples from secondary analyses I have conducted are presented here to illustrate approaches I have used in journal articles. I have published these secondary analyses using metaphorical analysis of my own datasets, and in each article, I chose a different way to present my results. In Chapter 8, on metaphor analysis, I described the research designs of these secondary qualitative analyses and their results. Here, I have provided the figures I used in publishing these studies. In the metaphor analysis of mothers' experiences of PTSD after birth (Beck, 2016), I created a word cloud of

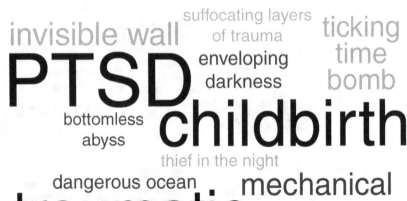

FIGURE 11.2 Word cloud of PTSD after birth metaphors.
Reprinted with permission from Beck (2016, p. 79).

the nine metaphors that emerged. In this word cloud the larger the named metaphor the more frequently it was used by the women in their narratives (Figure 11.2).

Eight metaphors were identified in my secondary analysis of mothers' descriptions of the anniversaries of their traumatic childbirth (Beck, 2017a). Charteris-Black (2012, p. 213) explained that "metaphors are like a series of brush-strokes so that no single metaphor adequately expresses the state." In publishing this secondary analysis, I created a figure of an easel, and on it were a series of brushstrokes, each one a different metaphor for the anniversary of birth trauma. Placement of the brushstrokes were organized in order of frequency of the use of the metaphors in the women's narratives. Those metaphors at the top of the easel were expressed more frequently than those at the bottom (Figure 11.3).

In my secondary qualitative analysis of the obstacle nightmare of shoulder dystocia, I created a table to compare the findings from two of the datasets I combined: one of the mothers' experiences and one of labor and delivery nurses' experiences (Table 11.2) (Beck, 2013). This side by side placement of quotes from the primary studies illustrated the striking similarity of both mothers' and nurses' perspectives on the harrowing experience of shoulder dystocia births. In my secondary analysis of metaphors mothers used to describe their experiences caring for their children with obstetric brachial plexus injuries (Beck, 2017b), I used images to illustrate each of the seven metaphors (Figure 11.4).

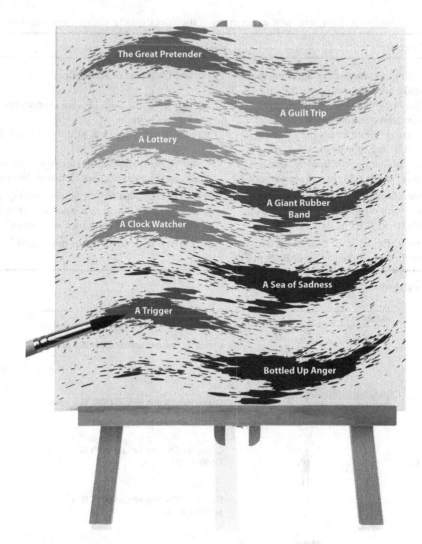

FIGURE 11.3 Eight metaphors of the anniversary of birth trauma.
Reprinted with permission from Beck (2017a, p. 223).

In summary, guidelines for publishing secondary qualitative analyses were explained. An outline for the structure for a journal article reporting secondary qualitative analysis was provided. Strategies to handle the challenges of writing this type of article were shared. Examples of figures and tables I have created and used in some of my published secondary qualitative analyses have been included as illustrations. In Chapter 12, the results of a literature review of secondary qualitative analyses conducted in one discipline, that is, nursing, are shared to identify the trends and methodologies used in these studies.

TABLE 11.2 Comparison of the traumatic experiences of shoulder dystocia: the obstetric nightmare

Mothers' Perspectives	Nurses' Perspectives
"The labor felt like I was assaulted for a prolonged time and like my child was assaulted at birth."	"I felt like I was part of a gang rape."
"If only I could have fought back then, but I was in a helpless position myself."	"I felt helpless at the birth because everything we tried didn't work."
"I was screaming 'Please let my baby be okay, please God let my baby be okay'."	"I was silently praying God, please save this baby."
"I never got congratulated when my baby was born. I wasn't even told there was an injury."	"The baby's head delivered and then there was silence. The nurses in the room gave each other 'the look'."
"The people who harm your baby for life just walk away with no apology and often no support." (Beck, 2009, p. 241)	"Feelings of regret that we (the nurses) didn't speak up. Scared because we were concerned about this baby prognosis, if it would come back as a lawsuit."
"I almost feel as if a part of me died on the day I gave birth. Isn't that ironic?" (Beck, 2009, p. 240)	"Immediately I felt numb. I was in shocked."

Reprinted with permission from Beck (2013, p. 36).

Metaphor #		Metaphor
1.	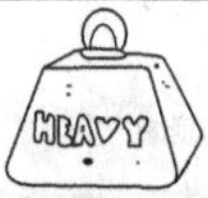	Caring for Children with an OBPI **IS** a heavy weight
2.	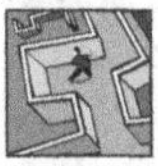	Caring for Children with an OBPI **IS** a maze
3.		Caring for Children with an OBPI **IS** a juggling act
4.	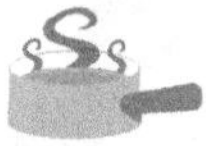	Caring for Children with an OBPI **IS** a simmering pot
5.	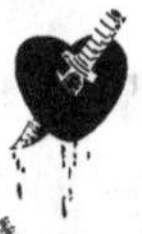	Caring for Children with an OBPI **IS** a dagger to the heart
6.	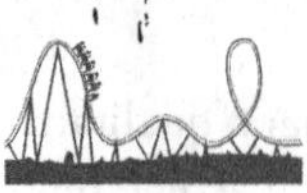	Caring for Children with an OBPI **IS** a roller-coaster
7.	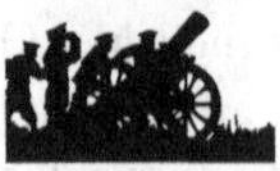	Caring for Children with an OBPI **IS** a constant battle

FIGURE 11.4 Seven metaphors in mothers' experiences caring for their children with obstetric brachial plexus injuries.

Reprinted with permission from Beck (2017b, p. 60).

References

Beck, C. T. (2009). The arm: There is no escaping the reality for mothers caring for their children with obstetric brachial plexus injuries. *Nursing Research, 58,* 237–245.

Beck, C. T. (2013). The obstetric nightmare of shoulder dystocia: A tale from two perspectives. *MCN: The American Journal of Maternal Child Nursing, 38,* 34–40.

Beck, C. T. (2016). Posttraumatic stress disorder after birth: A metaphorical analysis. *MCN: American Journal of Maternal Child Nursing, 41,* 76–83.

Beck, C. T. (2017a). The anniversary of birth trauma: A metaphor analysis. *The Journal of Perinatal Education, 26,* 219–228.

Beck, C. T. (2017b). Caring for a child with an obstetric brachial plexus injury: A metaphor analysis. *Journal of Pediatric Nursing, 36,* 57–63.

Charteris-Black, J. (2012). Shattering the bell jar: Metaphor, gender, and depression. *Metaphor and Symbol, 27,* 199–216.

12

REVIEW OF SECONDARY QUALITATIVE ANALYSIS IN THE DISCIPLINE OF NURSING

Heaton (2000) reviewed 65 secondary qualitative analyses in the area of social and health-care research to determine how this methodology was used in practice. Almost two decades later, I conducted a review of secondary qualitative analysis in one discipline, nursing, to describe existing practices. This is the focus of Chapter 12.

The purpose of this literature review was to:

- Assess the current state of the nursing discipline's use of secondary qualitative data analysis
- Identify the methodological aspects of these studies
- Make suggestions for future development of secondary qualitative analysis for researchers as they design, conduct, and publish these studies

Search strategy

The following databases were searched: Cinahl, PubMed, Scopus, and PsycINFO. No limits were put on how early the article had been published. Databases were searched through December 2017. Inclusion criteria were: English language, peer review journal, qualitative, first author a nurse, and secondary analysis. Examples of key words used were secondary analysis, secondary data analysis, qualitative, reuse, and nursing. Subject headings such as MeSH terms in Medline were entered. Boolean operators and wildcard and truncation symbols were also used, such as nurs*.

Abstracts were read and complete articles were printed if they met all the inclusion criteria. Frequent reasons for excluding articles were that they were qualitative systematic reviews or mixed methods studies, or that the term "secondary" was in the title, such as in secondary progressive multiple sclerosis, but not secondary qualitative analysis. In addition, in a number of studies qualitative content analysis was used to analyze the data but these studies were not secondary analyses.

Procedure

Once a decision was made that the article met all the inclusion criteria for this literature review, the Secondary Qualitative Data Analysis Codebook (Appendix A) was completed independently by myself and by my graduate assistant, Julia McNeil, who is a PhD student in nursing at the University of Connecticut. After completing the codebook for all the articles, we met to compare our findings. When we disagreed on a code for a variable, we discussed it until a consensus was reached. Our interrater reliability for the variables in the codebook ranged from 83%, for the variable of secondary analyst's relationship to the primary study, to 100%, for variables such as the country of the secondary analyst and clinical specialty. Nurse researchers from 20 different countries were represented in this review.

Results

From these databases, 274 secondary qualitative analyses conducted by nurse researchers were located. The earliest study was published in 1988. Two studies were published in the 1980s, 27 studies in the decade of the 1990s. Between the years 2000 and 2009, 84 secondary qualitative analyses were published, followed by 161 studies between the years 2010 and 2017. Each subsequent decade has seen at least a doubling in the number of these analyses being published.

Nurse researchers from which countries are leading in conducting these analyses? The top five countries were the United States ($n = 153$), Canada ($n = 61$), the United Kingdom ($n = 16$), Australia ($n = 12$), and Sweden ($n = 11$). Over half of the studies (56%) were conducted by U.S. researchers. The other countries, where between 1 and 4 secondary qualitative analyses had been published, included Denmark, New Zealand, China, Norway, South Africa, Slovenia, South Korea, Greece, Taiwan, Philippines, Pakistan, Switzerland, Israel, Spain, and Finland.

In Chapter 6, the different typologies of secondary qualitative data analyses were described. In this review of published analyses in nursing, only 68 of the 274 (24.8%) studies identified the typology that was used (Figure 12.1). Of these 68 studies, Thorne's typology was the most frequently cited one, followed by Heaton's, and then Hinds et al.'s. When looking at the studies citing Thorne's typology, analytic expansion was identified most often. Regarding Heaton's approach, supra analysis was most frequently cited as the type used. In Hinds and colleagues' typology, one study identified using a unit of analysis that differed from the original study, one used a subset of cases for a more focused analysis, and one reanalyzing all or part of the dataset focusing on a concept not specifically addressed in the original study. In the next section the description of the primary studies is first presented followed by the secondary analysis studies in this review from the discipline of nursing.

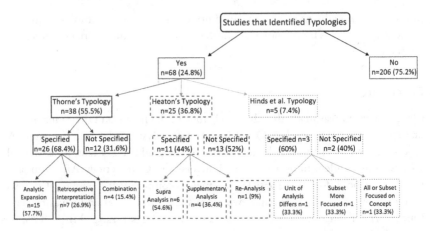

FIGURE 12.1 Secondary qualitative analysis typologies.

Primary studies

Research designs

Regarding the research designs the top five in order of frequency were descriptive qualitative ($n = 85$), mixed methods ($n = 56$), grounded theory ($n = 37$), phenomenology ($n = 25$), and ethnography ($n = 14$). Examples of other lesser used research designs were narrative analysis, focus groups, and interpretive description.

Sample size

The sample size of the primary studies had a wide range from 6 to 9915 (Mean = 165, SD = 672.12) with a median of 41.

Data collection method

When focusing on the primary data collection method, interviews were used most frequently ($n = 122$). Combinations of methods were also frequently cited such as focus groups, videotaping, journals, and written stories.

Data analysis

Turning to how data in the primary studies were analyzed, general thematic analysis ($n = 95$) was most frequently chosen, followed by a combination of methods ($n = 67$), then constant comparative method ($n = 38$) and phenomenological analyses ($n = 27$). Other lesser utilized methods included narrative analysis and interpretive description.

Secondary studies

Datasets

Out of the 274 studies in this review from the discipline of nursing, 144 (52.6%) studies incorporated the entire primary dataset, while 128 (46.7%) used a subset. Two studies used a combination of both an entire dataset plus a subset from another primary study. When considering the number of primary datasets used in the secondary qualitative analyses, 191 (69.7%) used one primary dataset while 74 (27%) utilized multiple primary datasets. In nine studies (3.2%) a primary dataset plus new supplementary data were used.

Secondary analyst's relationship to the primary research

In Table 12.1 are listed the variety of ways the secondary analysts were related to the original dataset. This variable had the lowest interrater reliability (83%) when my graduate assistant and I independently coded this variable. In 23 studies it was not clear at all who had conducted the original study. Other studies needed our detective work in examining reference lists in the articles and at times needing to obtain the primary study's publication to try and determine if the secondary analyst had been involved in the original study at all. In this review, these relationships were divided into two main categories. In the first one the secondary

TABLE 12.1 Secondary analyst's relationship to the primary research

Relationship	N	%
Original researcher		
Original researcher(s) reanalyze one primary dataset	44	16.1
Original researcher(s) reanalyze multiple datasets	16	5.8
Original researcher(s) reanalyze primary dataset(s) with new author(s)	81	29.6
Original researcher(s) reanalyze primary dataset(s) plus collect new supplementary data	5	1.8
Original researcher(s) reanalyze datasets with new additional authors plus collect new supplementary data	4	1.5
Multiple original researchers combine their datasets and reanalyze them together	17	6.2
Multiple original researchers combine their datasets and reanalyze with new additional authors	10	3.6
Secondary analyst		
Secondary analyst(s) with no previous involvement collaborate with original researcher(s)	57	20.8
Secondary analyst(s) with no previous involvement alone with original dataset	7	2.6
Secondary analyst(s) with prior involvement with original dataset collaborating with original researcher	8	2.9
Secondary analyst(s) with no prior involvement with original dataset not collaborating with original researcher(s)	2	0.7

analysts also had been the primary researchers in the original study. The second main category focused on secondary analysts who had not been the primary researchers of the original dataset.

There were seven different ways primary researchers were involved in the secondary qualitative analyses. The most frequent relationship occurred when primary researchers reanalyzed their own original datasets with additional new researchers (n = 81). In 44 studies primary researchers alone reanalyzed one of their original datasets. In 16 studies primary researchers alone combined their multiple datasets together and reanalyzed them. In four studies the primary researchers reused their own datasets with additional new researchers plus collected new supplementary data. Multiple primary researchers combined their datasets and reanalyzed them together in 17 studies while in 10 studies multiple primary researchers combined and reanalyzed their datasets with additional new researchers.

When secondary analysts were first authors of the secondary qualitative analyses, four different relationships with the original dataset were identified. The most frequent relationship (n = 57) occurred when the secondary analyst had no previous involvement with the original dataset but collaborated with the primary researcher. Then in 10 studies, the secondary analyst did have prior involvement with the original dataset and collaborated with the primary researcher. In seven studies, the secondary analyst had no previous involvement with the original dataset and worked alone in the secondary analysis.

Consultation with the primary researcher

Whether secondary analysts consulted with the primary researchers was another variable coded in this literature review. In the majority of studies 64% (n = 175) consultation with the primary researcher was not necessary since the primary researcher was part of the secondary analysis team. In a quarter of the studies (n = 69) the secondary analyst did consult with the primary researcher. In 30 studies (11%), the secondary analysts did not specify whether they consulted with the primary researcher.

Ethical approval

It was stated in all the articles that Institutional Review Board (IRB) approval had been obtained to conduct the primary studies. However, in only 93 studies (33%) was it specifically stated that ethical approval had been obtained for the secondary analysis.

Sample size

The sample size of the primary studies also had a wide range from 2 to 3319 (Mean = 73.74, SD = 222.38) with a median of 30.

Data sources

The most frequently used data source was interview transcripts ($n = 187$), followed by a combination of data sources ($n = 50$), such as field notes and interviews. In third place ($n = 13$) were answers to open-ended questions. Additional sources of data used less frequently included online forum posts, stories, and journals.

Data analysis

Out of the 274 studies general thematic analysis was used most often ($n = 95$), content analysis ($n = 92$) was second in frequency, constant comparative method was in third place ($n = 30$), phenomenological analysis ($n = 16$) in fourth, and interpretive description ($n = 12$) took fifth place. Other additional data analysis techniques utilized less frequently included metaphor analysis, discourse analysis, and narrative analysis.

Outcomes

When looking at the results of the secondary qualitative analyses in this nursing review, in 163 (60%) studies the outcomes were in the form of themes. In second place were categories ($n = 74$, 27%), and in third place concepts were the outcome ($n = 11$, 4%). Other less common outcomes included models, grounded theory, and metaphors.

Discussion

Heaton's (2000) review of qualitative secondary data analyses in social and health-care research has been the only one prior to this review in nursing. Where it was possible, a comparison of some characteristics was made between these two reviews. Even though two decades had passed between these two reviews, there were some similarities noted. For example, in Heaton's review almost 50% of the secondary analytic studies reused the entire original dataset and 50% reused only a subset. In this current nursing review, only in slightly more than half (52.6%) was the entire primary dataset reused versus 46.7% that reused only subsets. Heaton reported that in 74% of the secondary analytic studies a single dataset was reanalyzed while 26% reused two or more datasets. For this nursing review, 69.2% of the studies reused one primary dataset, while 27% utilized multiple original datasets. In both reviews interviews were the most frequently used data collection method. Regarding studies where the secondary analysts had no previous involvement with the primary research, Heaton reported 14%, while in this current review, it was 2.5%. In 23 studies in the nursing review, however, the relationship between the secondary analyst and the primary study was not clear, so this number of no prior involvement could be higher. In both reviews there was a low percentage of secondary analyses where the secondary analyst collected new data to add to the primary dataset. Heaton identified 14% of the studies while in only 3% of the nursing studies were additional data collected to supplement the original study.

In the remainder of this chapter, some methodological and ethical issues are reflected on and recommendations made based on this nursing review. Secondary qualitative analysis certainly has been on the upswing in nursing. From 1988 when the first analysis was published, the number of studies has doubled in each of the successive decades. What seemed to be helping this rise in secondary qualitative analyses is the growing popularity of mixed methods research. Out of the 274 studies in this review, 70 studies (25.5%) had mixed methods as the research design in the primary study. Data from the qualitative strand of the mixed methods studies were used in these secondary qualitative analyses.

Take always from this literature review of one discipline are recommendations not only for nurse researchers but for all secondary analysts as they design, conduct, and publish their studies. It needs to be clearly stated in the articles that ethical approval had been obtained to conduct the secondary qualitative analysis. It is not enough to state that approval had been obtained for the primary study. Description of how and when the approval was obtained for the secondary analysis should be addressed. For example, did the informed consent for the primary study also include approval for further use of the data by the research team and other researchers?

Secondary analysts need to identify the typology of secondary qualitative analysis they used. Was it Thorne's, Heaton's, or Hinds and colleagues' typology? It is not enough to state the chosen typology. Secondary analysts then need to go one step further and state what type of analysis in that typology was used. For example, if Heaton's typology was utilized, did the secondary analysts use supra analysis, supplementary analysis, or reanalysis?

Regarding how the secondary research reanalyzed the primary dataset, if thematic analysis was used, it strengthens the study if a specific method for developing the themes is cited and used rather than just stating a generic thematic analysis. Attention needs to also be paid to clearly describing the methodology used in the primary study. For instance, what were the research questions? Who was the primary researcher? In this literature review, at times, it was not clear who exactly had conducted the primary study. Therefore, it was not possible to determine the relationship between the primary and secondary researchers.

In regards to the secondary analysts, it should be specified if they had collaborated in some way in the primary study or not. The secondary analysts' relationship to the original dataset is important and should be easily identified by the readers of the secondary analysis. If the secondary analysts were not involved in the primary studies, it needs to be clear if they consulted with the primary researcher while they were reanalyzing the original dataset.

In summary, the results of a review of 274 secondary qualitative data analyses conducted in the discipline of nursing were presented. Characteristics of the studies such as, the country of the first author, year published, and typology of secondary qualitative analysis were identified. Methodological features of both the primary and secondary studies were coded. Trends and limitations in the reporting of these research designs were noted and recommendations made. In the final chapter, Chapter 13, the future of secondary qualitative data analysis is envisioned and recommendations made.

Reference

Heaton, J. (2000). *Secondary analysis of qualitative data: A review of the literature*. York, England: Social Policy Research Unit (SPRU), University of York.

13

WHAT IS AROUND THE CORNER FOR SECONDARY QUALITATIVE DATA ANALYSIS?

The future looks bright and exciting for secondary qualitative analysis. The reuse of qualitative datasets will increase as more qualitative data archives become available and more funders require the availability of sharing qualitative findings for reuse in order to maximize the value of the data for the public good. Also, as more qualitative researchers obtain consent for secondary analysis right at the start of their primary studies, some of the ethical roadblocks will be removed. As more secondary qualitative analyses are published, researchers will become aware of this method's many valuable uses, such as theory development, metaphor analysis, and health services policy, to name a few. Secondary qualitative data analysis can also help in the health-care arena to expedite the translation of qualitative findings to provide evidence-based practice to improve patient care.

Some lesser known purposes of secondary qualitative analysis will come more into the forefront. Ziebland and Hunt (2014) argued that due to financial or time constraints policy makers often cannot conduct a new study to help informed policy. It is important for the development of health services policy that the voices and experiences of patients are included as valuable evidence. This is where secondary qualitative analysis can be used to bring patients' experiences to the center of health policy. Otherwise, the exclusion of patients' experiences can silence or marginalize these voices in policy formation.

Theory development is another area that attention has not been focused on as a valuable option for reuse of qualitative datasets. Morse (2018) warns us that qualitative researchers have only partially fulfilled the promise of developing concepts and theories. Secondary qualitative analysis can help make a major contribution to knowledge development. Theoretical coalescence is one method that researchers can use to reanalyze their datasets to develop qualitative theory or conduct a concept analysis.

Metaphor analysis is central to providing understanding. When a metaphor is linked to its experiential basis that is when it is able to deepen understanding and capture the essence of an experience (Lakoff & Johnson, 1980). In the health-care sciences, metaphors can help patients explain what they are experiencing in their everyday lives with their illnesses and communicate more effectively with clinicians in ways they cannot with unfamiliar medical terminology. Qualitative researchers will soon learn how much fun metaphor analysis is as a type of sec-ondary qualitative analysis. Not every qualitative dataset, however, will have enough metaphors to reanalyze, but when it does enjoy the process.

Recommendations for ethical issues

Preplanning for reuse of data is best done during the initial consent process. Multiple layers of consent should be included in an informed consent. First the person gives consent to participate in the primary study. Next, the option of giving permission for the primary researcher to reuse the data is necessary. Another option is to give participants a choice of letting other researchers than the primary one reuse their data. Last is the option of whether or not the participant gives permission to archive their data. During the initial consent process options for archiving data also need to be explained to the participant such as, who will have access to their data, where will the data be stored, and options for limiting access to their data.

Recommendations for qualitative data archiving

Qualitative researchers should contact institutional and repository representa-tives at the earliest stages of planning. Guidelines for the specific archive can then be followed to make appropriate preparations for data archiving and sharing. Primary researchers need to pay attention to what they will include in their metadata for sharing. Qualitative archives can increase the opportunities for cross-country comparisons. What would be helpful is a central website where all qualitative data archives' contact information is listed.

Recommendations for publication

In publishing their secondary qualitative analyses, researchers need to be atten-tive to describing the specifics of not only their secondary analyses but also the primary studies. Details of the original study from which the qualitative dataset comes from need to be specified in the article. Details such as, the original research questions, sample size, and primary researchers involved in the study are important to share with the readers. In describing the secondary analysis researchers need to pay more attention to their methodology such as, whose typology they used and from that typology what specific type of analysis did they use. For example, did they use Thorne's (2013) typology and specifically analytic expansion? Researchers also need to make clear the secondary analyst's relationship to the primary study.

Recommendations for education

Faculty involved in teaching qualitative research methods courses in PhD programs need to include content on secondary qualitative data analysis in their syllabi. Not only content on this type of analysis but also hands-on practice reusing a qualitative dataset is needed in order to prepare our next generation of qualitative researchers. With the upswing in the number of mixed methods studies, more datasets from the qualitative strands will be available for reuse. Faculty teaching mixed methods research courses need to alert their students of this valuable option with the qualitative strands. If faculty do not have their own qualitative datasets to use in their courses, some qualitative data archives, as identified in Chapter 7, have datasets that are available for students to use to practice reusing qualitative datasets. Research internships for PhD students with secondary qualitative data analysis should be made available. In qualitative research methods courses, time needs to be set aside also for critiquing published secondary qualitative analyses. Guidelines for writing and publishing a secondary qualitative analysis also need to be taught in these courses.

References

Lakoff, G., & Johnson, M. (1980). *Metaphors we live by.* Chicago, IL: University of Chicago Press.

Morse, J. M. (2018). Theoretical coalescence: A method to develop qualitative theory: The example of enduring. *Nursing Research, 67,* 177–187.

Thorne, S. (2013). Secondary qualitative data analysis. In C. T. Beck (Ed.), *Routledge international handbook of qualitative nursing research* (pp. 393–416). New York: Routledge.

Ziebland, S., & Hunt, K. (2014). Using secondary analysis of qualitative data of patient experiences of healthcare to inform health services research and policy. *Journal of Health Services Research & Policy, 19,* 177–182.

APPENDIX A

GUIDANCE ON SECONDARY ANALYSIS OF EXISTING DATA SETS

The University of Connecticut Institutional Review Board (IRB) recognizes that some research projects involving existing data sets and archives may not meet the definition of "human subjects" research requiring IRB review; some may meet definitions of research that is exempt from the federal regulations at 45 CFR part 46; and some may require IRB review. This document is intended to provide guidance on IRB policies and procedures and to reduce burdens associated with IRB review for investigators whose research involves only the analysis of existing data sets and archives. The IRB acknowledges the guidance document prepared by the University of Chicago Social and Behavioral Sciences IRB as the model for this Guidance.

Although projects that only involve secondary data analysis do not involve interactions or interventions with humans, they may still require IRB review, because the definition of "human subject" at 45 CFR 46.102(f) includes living individuals *about whom an investigator obtains identifiable private information for research purposes.*

1. When does secondary use of existing data *not* require IRB review?

In general, the secondary analysis of existing data does not require IRB review when it does not fall within the regulatory definition of research involving human subjects.

Public use data sets

Public use data sets are prepared with the intent of making them available for the public. The data available to the public are not individually identifiable and therefore analysis would not involve human subjects. The IRB recognizes that the analysis of de-identified, publicly available data does not constitute human subjects research as defined at 45 CFR 46.102 and that it does not require IRB review. The IRB no longer requires the registration or review of studies involving the analysis of public use data sets **unless** a project merges multiple data sets and in so doing enables the identification of individuals whose data are analyzed. An IRB review may be required for a research study that relies exclusively on secondary use of anonymous information BUT records data linkage or disseminates results in such a way that it generates identifiable information.

In addition to being identifiable, existing data must include "private information" in order to constitute research involving human subjects. Private information is defined as information which has been provided for specific purposes by an individual and which the individual can reasonably expect will not be made public (e.g., a medical or school record). For example, a study involving only analysis of the published salaries and benefits of university presidents would not need IRB review since this information is not private.

De-identified data

If a dataset has been stripped of all identifying information and there is no way it could be linked back to the subjects from whom it was originally collected (through a key to a coding system or by other means), its subsequent use by the Principal Investigator or by another researcher would not constitute human subjects research, since the data are no longer identifiable. "Identifiable" means the identity of the subject is known or may be readily ascertained by the investigator or associated with the information. In general, information is considered to be identifiable when it can be linked to specific individuals by the researcher either directly or indirectly through coding systems, or when characteristics of the information obtained are such that a reasonably knowledgeable person could ascertain the identities of individuals. Even though a dataset has been stripped of direct identifiers (e.g., names, addresses, student ID numbers, etc.), it may still be possible to identify an individual through a combination of other characteristics (e.g., age, gender, ethnicity, place of employment).

Example: Many student research projects involve secondary analysis of data that belongs to, or was initially collected by, their faculty advisor or another investigator. If the student is provided with a de-identified, non-coded data set, the use of the data does not constitute research with human subjects because there is no interaction with any individual and no identifiable private information will be used.

Coded data: Secondary analysis of coded private information is not considered to be research involving human subjects and would not require IRB review **IF** the investigator(s) cannot readily ascertain the identity of the individuals to whom the coded private information pertains as a result of one of the following circumstances:

1. The investigators and the holder of the key have entered into an agreement prohibiting the release of the key to the investigators under any

circumstances, until the individuals are deceased (HHS regulations for human subjects research do not require the IRB to review and approve this agreement);

2.   There are IRB-approved written policies and operating procedures for a repository or data management center that prohibit the release of the key to the investigator under any circumstances, until the individuals are deceased; or

3.   There are other legal requirements prohibiting the release of the key to the investigators, until the individuals are deceased.

For more information on when analysis of coded data is or is not human subjects research, see the **HHS Office for Human Research Protections Guidance on Research Involving Coded Private Information or Biological Specimens** at http://www.hhs.gov/ohrp/policy/cdebiol.html.

Note: If a student is analyzing *coded data* from a faculty advisor/sponsor who retains a key, this would be human subjects research, because the faculty advisor is considered an investigator on the student's protocol, and can readily ascertain the identity of the subjects since he/she holds the key to the coded data. If the student's work fits within the scope of the initial protocol from which the dataset originates, the faculty advisor (or investigator who holds the dataset) may wish to consider adding the student and his/her work to the original protocol by means of an amendment application rather than having the student submit a new application for review.

Example: Researcher B plans to examine the relationships between attention deficit hyperactivity disorder (ADHD), oppositional defiance disorder, and teen drug abuse using data collected by Agencies I, II, and III that work with "at risk" youth. The data will be coded and the agencies have entered into an agreement prohibiting release of the key to the researcher that could connect the data with identifiers. The use of the data would not constitute research with human subjects.

If the IRB determines that the project does not constitute human subjects research, the IRB will notify the investigator. If the IRB determines that the project does involve human subjects research, the investigator will be asked to submit a protocol for consideration by the IRB.

2. When is the secondary use of existing data exempt?

There are six categories of research activities involving human subjects that may be exempt from the requirements of the federal regulations on human subjects research protections (45 CFR 46.101(2)(b)). However, only one exemption category (Category 4) applies specifically to existing data. If research is found to be exempt, it need not receive full or expedited review. In order to qualify for an exempt determination, an IRB-5 application must be submitted in InfoEd for IRB review.

Research involving collection or study of existing data, documents, and records can be exempted under Category 4 of the federal regulations if: (i) the sources of such data are publicly available; or (ii) the information is recorded by the investigator in such a manner that subjects cannot be identified, directly or through identifiers linked to the subjects.

The latter condition of this category applies in cases where the investigators initially have access to identifiable private information but abstract the data needed for the research in such a way that the information can no longer be connected to the identity of the subjects. This means that the abstracted data set does not include **direct identifiers** (names, social security numbers, addresses, phone numbers, etc.) **or indirect identifiers** (codes or pseudonyms that are linked to the subject's identity). Furthermore, it must not be possible to identify subjects by combining a number of characteristics (e.g., date of birth, gender, position, and place of employment). This is especially relevant in smaller datasets, where the population is confined to a limited subject pool.

The following do *not* qualify for exemption: Research involving prisoners, and FDA-regulated research.

Example: Student A will be given access to data from her faculty advisor's health survey research project. The data consists of coded survey responses, and the advisor will retain a key that would link the data to identifiers. The student will extract the information she needs for her project without including any identifying information and without retaining the code. The use of the data does constitute research with human subjects because the initial data set is identifiable (albeit through a coding system); however, it would qualify for exempt status.

3. When does the secondary use of existing data require expedited or full board review?

If secondary analysis of existing data does involve research with human subjects and does not qualify for exempt status as explained above, the project must be reviewed either through expedited procedures or by the full (convened) IRB, and an IRB-1 protocol application must be submitted in InfoEd for IRB review.

Consent: Researchers using data previously collected under another study should consider whether the currently proposed research is a "compatible use" with what subjects agreed to in the original consent form. For non-exempt projects, a consent process description or justification for a waiver must be included in the research protocol.

The IRB may require that informed consent for secondary analysis be obtained from subjects whose data will be accessed.

Alternatively, the IRB can consider a request for a waiver of one or more elements of informed consent under 45 CFR 46.116(d). In order to approve such waiver, the IRB must first be satisfied that the research:

1. presents minimal risk (no risks of harm, considering probability and magnitude, greater than those ordinarily encountered in daily life or during the performance of routine examinations or tests); and

2. the waiver or alteration will not adversely affect the rights and welfare of the subjects; and
3. the research could not practicably be carried out without the waiver or alteration; and
4. whenever appropriate, the subjects will be provided with additional pertinent information after participation.

"Restricted Use Data": Certain agencies and research organizations release files to researchers with specific restrictions regarding their use and storage. These restrictions are typically described in a data use or restricted use data agreement the organization requires be signed in order to receive the data. The records frequently contain identifiers or extensive variables that combined might enable identification, even though this is not the intent of the researcher. Research using these data sets requires expedited or full board level review. Note that the data use or restricted use data agreement must be reviewed by Sponsored Programs Services (SPS) prior to institutional approval. The IRB will not approve the study until the agreement receives approval by SPS. The protocol may be submitted to the IRB at the same time the agreement is submitted to SPS.

Examples

1. Student C will be given access to coded mental health assessments from his faculty advisor's research project. The student plans to analyze the data with a code attached to each record, and the advisor will retain a key to the code that would link the data to identifiers. The use of the data does constitute research with human subjects and does not qualify for exempt status since subjects can be identified. This student project would require an IRB-1 protocol application to be submitted in InfoEd for expedited or full board review by the IRB.

    Note: As previously noted, if the student's work fits within the scope of the initial protocol from which the dataset originates, the faculty advisor (or investigator who holds the dataset) may wish to consider adding the student and his/her work to the original protocol by means of an amendment application rather than having the student submit a new application for expedited or full board review.

2. Student D is applying to the National Center for Health Statistics for use of data from the National Health and Nutrition Examination Survey that includes geographic identifiers and date of examination. The analysis of this restricted use data would require IRB-1 protocol application to be submitted in InfoEd for expedited or full board review by the IRB.

Note: The materials presented here are compiled from a mix of the Office for Human Research Protections (OHRP) and other Universities' online sources.
Reprinted with permission for the University of Connecticut.

APPENDIX B

INFORMED CONSENT FOR PARTICIPATION IN A RESEARCH STUDY

Principal Investigator: Cheryl Tatano Beck, DNSc, CNM, FAAN
Study Title: Impact of Traumatic Childbirth on Mothers' Experiences Caring for Their Children

Introduction

You are invited to participate in a research study so that we can better understand the impact of traumatic childbirth on mothers' experiences interacting with and caring for their infants and older children.

Why is this study being done?

For decades now researchers have studied the long term effects that postpartum depression can have on mother-infant interactions and child development. Much less attention has focused on the possible effects of posttraumatic stress on mother-infant interaction and attachment and children's emotional and cognitive development. The purpose of this study is to help understand the experiences of mothers who have had a traumatic birth and how this may impact their interactions with their infants and older children.

What are the study procedures? What will I be asked to do?

If you agree to take part in this survey via electronic survey you will be asked to complete (1) a participant Profile Form which includes questions about yourself such as your age, education, and type of birth, and (2) to describe in as much detail as you wish your experiences of caring for and interacting with your infant and any older children you may have. Depending on how in depth you write about your experiences, participation in the study could take between 30- 60 minutes.

What are the risks or inconveniences of the study?

We believe there are no known risks associated with this research study; however, if you become anxious remembering your traumatic childbirth please know you can stop participating in the study. You do not have to complete the study. One possible inconvenience to you may be the time it takes to complete this survey.

What are the benefits of the study?

You may not directly benefit from this research; however, we hope your participation in this survey will help health care professionals provide better care to mothers who have experienced a traumatic childbirth.

Will I receive payment for participation? Are there costs to participate?

There are no costs and you will not be paid to be in this study.

How will my personal information be protected?

The following procedures will be used to protect the confidentiality of your data. The researchers will keep all study records indefinitely in a locked secure location. Research records will be labeled with a code. The code will be derived from a sequential 3 digit number that reflects how many people have enrolled in the study. A master key that links names and codes will be maintained in a separate and secure location. All electronic files (e.g., database, spreadsheet, etc.) will be password protected. Any computer hosting such files will also have password protection to prevent access by unauthorized users. Only the members of the research staff will have access to the passwords. Data that will be shared with others will be coded as described above to protect your identity. Study records will be kept indefinitely once the data have been stripped of identifiable information. At the conclusion of this study, the researchers may publish their findings. Information will be presented in summary format and you will not be identified in any publications or presentations.

"We will do our best to protect the confidentiality of the information we gather from you but we cannot guarantee 100% confidentiality. Your confidentiality will be maintained to the degree permitted by the technology used. Specifically, no guarantees can be made regarding the interception of data sent via the Internet by any third parties." **Data that we collect from you may be shared with other researchers in the future, but only after your name and all identifying information have been removed.**

You should also know that the UConn Institutional Review Board (IRB) and Research Compliance Services may inspect study records as part of its auditing program, but these reviews will only focus on the researchers and not on your responses or involvement. The IRB is a group of people who review research studies to protect the rights and welfare of research participants.

Can I stop being in the study and what are my rights?

You do not have to be in this study if you do not want to. If you agree to be in the study, but later change your mind, you may drop out at any time. There are no penalties or consequences of any kind if you decide that you do not want to participate.

Whom do I contact if I have questions about the study?

Take as long as you like before you make a decision. We will be happy to answer any question you have about this study. If you have further questions about this project or if you have a research-related problem, you may contact the Principal Investigator (Dr. Cheryl Beck, 860-486-0547). If you have any questions concerning your rights as a research subject, you may contact the University of Connecticut Institutional Review Board (IRB) at 860-486-8802.

Documentation of Consent:

I have read this form and decided that I will participate in the project described above. Its general purposes, the particulars of involvement and possible risks and inconveniences have been explained to my satisfaction. I understand that I can withdraw at any time. My signature also indicates that I have received a copy of this consent form.

_____   _____   _____
Participant Signature: Print Name: Date:

_____   _____   _____
Signature of Person   Print Name: Date:

Obtaining Consent

APPENDIX C

SECONDARY QUALITATIVE DATA ANALYSIS CODEBOOK

ID number: _____

Reference (author/year published)

Clinical specialty		First author's country	
Clinical specialty	1. Nurses	First author's country	1. U.S.
	2. Nursing education		2. U.K.
	3. Palliative care		3. Canada
	4. Oncology		4. Sweden
	5. Obstetrics		5. Denmark
	6. Women's health/gynecology		6. China
	7. Pediatrics		7. Norway
	8. Medical surgical		8. South Africa
	9. Psych/mental health		9. Slovenia
	10. Gerontology		10. Australia
	11. Community health		11. New Zealand
	12. Other		12. Switzerland
	13. Combination		13. South Korea
			14. Greece
			15. Israel

16. Taiwan
17. Pakistan
18. Philippines
19. Spain
20. Finland

Primary study (research design)

1. Descriptive qualitative
2. Phenomenology
3. Grounded theory
4. Ethnography
5. Narrative analysis
6. Focus groups
7. Interpretive description
8. Mixed methods
9. RCT
10. Combination
11. Other
12. Discourse analysis

Primary study (data collection)

1. Interviews/audiotaped
2. Focus groups
3. Observation
4. Video taping
5. Internet
6. Logs/journals
7. Clinical/medical journals
8. Open-ended questions
9. Field notes
10. Written/oral stories
11. Questionnaires
12. Combination
13. Other

Sample size of primary study: _____

Primary study (or studies) data analysis technique

1. Content analysis
2. Phenomenological analysis
3. Constant comparative method GT
4. Metaphor analysis
5. Narrative analysis
6. Ethnographic approach
7. General qualitative/thematic analysis
8. Interpretive description
9. Quantitative
10. Combination
11. Other

Secondary analyst's relationship to primary research

Original researcher
1. Original researcher(s) reanalyze one primary dataset
2. Original researcher(s) reanalyze multiple datasets
3. Original researcher(s) reanalyze primary dataset(s) with new author(s)

4. Original researcher(s) reanalyze primary dataset(s) plus collect new supplementary data
5. Original researcher(s) reanalyze data set with new additional authors plus collect new supplementary data
6. Multiple original researchers combine their datasets and reanalyze them together
7. Multiple original researchers combine their datasets & reanalyze with new additional authors

Secondary analyst

8. Secondary analyst(s) with no previous involvement collaborate with original researcher(s)
9. Secondary analyst(s) with no previous involvement alone with original dataset
10. Secondary analyst(s) with prior involvement with original dataset collaborating with original researcher(s)
11. Secondary analyst(s) with prior involvement with original dataset not collaborating with original researcher(s)
12. Other
13. Not clear who conducted original study

Dataset used in secondary study	1. Entire primary dataset(s) 2. Sub-set(s) 3. Combination
Number of datasets used in secondary study	1. One primary dataset 2. Multiple primary datasets 3. Primary dataset plus new supplementary data
Type of research data used in secondary study	1. Interview transcripts 2. Audio recordings 3. Field notes 4. Emails 5. Observation 6. Video 7. Answers to open ended questions 8. Journals/ logs 9. Unsolicited comments in quantitative survey 10. Photo voice 11. Online forum posts 12. Stories 13. Questionnaire 14. Clinical/medical records 15. Combination 16. Other
Secondary study (or studies) data analysis technique	1. Content analysis 2. Phenomenological analysis 3. Constant comparative method (GT) 4. Narrative analysis

	5. Metaphor analysis
	6. Ethnographic
	7. General qualitative/thematic analysis
	8. Interpretive description
	9. Discourse analysis
	10. Combination
	11. Not specified
	12. Other
Consultation with primary researcher during secondary analysis	1. Yes 2. No 3. NA 4. Not specified

Sample size of secondary study: _____

Was ethical approval for secondary analysis specifically obtained?	1. Yes 2. No 3. Not specified
Type of secondary data analysis approach	1. Specified 2. Not specified
If yes, which specific approach?	1. Thorne 2. Heaton 3. Hinds, Vogel, & Clarke-Steffen 4. Other
Type of Thorne's secondary analysis approach	1. Analytic expansion 2. Retrospective interpretation 3. Armchair induction 4. Cross-validation 5. Amplified sampling 6. Not specified 7. Combination
Type of Heaton's secondary data analysis approach	1. Supra analysis 2. Supplementary analysis 3. Re-analysis 4. Amplified analysis 5. Assorted analysis 6. Not specified 7. Combination
Type of Hinds, Vogel & Clarke-Steffen secondary data analysis approach	1. Use a unit of analysis that differs from that used in primary study 2. Extract a subset of cases for a similar but more focused analysis relative to primary study 3. Reanalyze all or part of data set by focusing on a concept that was not specifically addressed in primary analysis 4. Using an existing data set as one data source while continuing to refine the study purpose, questions, & data collection processes. 5. Not specified

Outcome of secondary data analysis	1. Themes
	2. Categories/domains/patterns/issue/dimensions/types
	3. Grounded theory
	4. Concept analysis/concepts
	5. Model
	6. Narratives
	7. Metaphors
	8. Interpretative description
	9. Other

INDEX

Note: **Boldface** page numbers refer to tables; *italic* page numbers refer to figures.

Printed in the United States
by Baker & Taylor Publisher Services